Hematology

Editor

TERRY W. CAMPBELL

VETERINARY CLINICS OF NORTH AMERICA: EXOTIC ANIMAL PRACTICE

www.vetexotic.theclinics.com

Consulting Editor
AGNES E. RUPLEY

January 2015 • Volume 18 • Number 1

ELSEVIER

1600 John F. Kennedy Boulevard • Suite 1800 • Philadelphia, Pennsylvania, 19103-2899

http://www.vetexotic.theclinics.com

VETERINARY CLINICS OF NORTH AMERICA: EXOTIC ANIMAL PRACTICE Volume 18, Number 1
January 2015 ISSN 1094-9194, ISBN-13: 978-0-323-35598-8

Editor: Patrick Manley
Developmental Editor: Casey Jackson

Veterinary Clinics of North America: Exotic Animal Practice (ISSN 1094-9194) is published in January, May, and September by Elsevier, Inc., 360 Park Avenue South, New York, NY 10010-1710. Subscription prices are $255.00 per year for US individuals, $399.00 per year for US institutions, $130.00 per year for US students and residents, $305.00 per year for Canadian individuals, $482.00 per year for Canadian institutions, $340.00 per year for international individuals, $482.00 per year for international institutions and $165.00 per year for Canadian and foreign students/residents. To receive student/resident rate, orders must be accompanied by name of affiliated institution, date of term, and the *signature* of program/residency coordinator on institution letterhead. Orders will be billed at individual rate until proof of status is received. Foreign air speed delivery is included in all *Clinics* subscription prices. All prices are subject to change without notice. **POSTMASTER:** Send address changes to *Veterinary Clinics of North America: Exotic Animal Practice*, Elsevier Health Sciences Division, Subscription Customer Service, 3251 Riverport Lane, Maryland Heights, MO 63043. **Customer Service: Telephone: 1-800-654-2452** (U.S. and Canada); **1-314-447-8871** (outside U.S. and Canada). **Fax: 1-314-447-8029. E-mail: journalscustomerservice-usa@elsevier.com** (for print support); **journalsonlinesupport-usa@elsevier.com** (for online support).

Reprints. For copies of 100 or more of articles in this publication, please contact the Commercial Reprints Department, Elsevier Inc., 360 Park Avenue South, New York, New York 10010-1710. Tel.: 212-633-3874; Fax: 212-633-3820; E-mail: reprints@elsevier.com.

Veterinary Clinics of North America: Exotic Animal Practice is covered in *MEDLINE/PubMed (Index Medicus).*

Contributors

CONSULTING EDITOR

AGNES E. RUPLEY, DVM
Diplomate, American Board of Veterinary Practitioners–Avian Practice; Director and Chief Veterinarian, All Pets Medical & Laser Surgical Center, College Station, Texas

EDITOR

TERRY W. CAMPBELL, MS, DVM, PhD
Associate Professor, Department of Clinical Sciences, College of Veterinary Medicine and Biomedical Sciences, Colorado State University, Fort Collins, Colorado

AUTHORS

ANDREA A. BOHN, DVM, PhD
Diplomate, American College of Veterinary Pathologists; Associate Professor, Department of Microbiology, Immunology, and Pathology, College of Veterinary Medicine and Biomedical Sciences, Colorado State University, Fort Collins, Colorado

TERRY W. CAMPBELL, MS, DVM, PhD
Associate Professor, Department of Clinical Sciences, College of Veterinary Medicine and Biomedical Sciences, Colorado State University, Fort Collins, Colorado

CAROLYN CRAY, PhD
Professor of Clinical Pathology and Microbiology & Immunology, Division of Comparative Pathology, Department of Pathology, University of Miami Miller School of Medicine, Miami, Florida

BOB DONELEY, BVSc, FACVSc (Avian Health), CMAVA
Veterinary Medical Centre, School of Veterinary Science, University of Queensland, Gatton, Queensland, Australia

KRYSTAN R. GRANT, DVM
Department of Clinical Sciences, Colorado State University, Fort Collins, Colorado

MICHAEL P. JONES, DVM
Diplomate American Board of Veterinary Practitioners (Avian Practice), Associate Professor, Avian & Zoological Medicine, Department of Small Animal Clinical Sciences, University of Tennessee, College of Veterinary Medicine, Knoxville, Tennessee

ERIC KLAPHAKE, DVM
Diplomate, American College of Zoological Medicine; Diplomate, American Board of Veterinary Practitioners (Avian); Diplomate, American Board of Veterinary Practitioners (Reptile/Amphibian); Cheyenne Mountain Zoo, Colorado Springs, Colorado

NICOLE M. LINDSTROM, MS, DVM
Laboratory Animal Veterinary Program Specialist, Virginia Tech, Blacksburg, Virginia

DAVID M. MOORE, MS, DVM
Diplomate of the American College of Laboratory Animal Medicine; Associate Vice President for Research Compliance, Department of Biomedical Sciences and Pathobiology, North End Center, Virginia Tech, Blacksburg, Virginia

STEPHEN A. SMITH, MS, DVM, PhD
Professor of Aquatic, Wildlife and Pocket Pet Medicine, Department of Biomedical Sciences and Pathobiology (0442), Virginia-Maryland Regional College of Veterinary Medicine, Blacksburg, Virginia

JOHN M. SYKES IV, DVM
Diplomate, American College of Zoological Medicine; Senior Veterinarian, Zoological Health Program, Wildlife Conservation Society, Bronx Zoo, Bronx, New York

LINDA VAP, DVM
Diplomate, American College of Veterinary Pathologists; Assistant Professor, Department of Microbiology, Immunology, and Pathology, College of Veterinary Medicine and Biomedical Sciences, Colorado State University, Fort Collins, Colorado

ELIZABETH G. WELLES, DVM, PhD
Diplomate, American College of Veterinary Pathologists; Professor, Department of Pathobiology, Auburn University, Auburn, Alabama

KURT ZIMMERMAN, DVM, PhD
Diplomate, American College of Veterinary Pathologists; Associate Professor of Clinical and Anatomical Pathology, Department of Biomedical Sciences and Pathobiology (0442), Virginia-Maryland Regional College of Veterinary Medicine, Blacksburg, Virginia

Contents

Pet ferrets are presented to veterinary clinics for routine care and treatment of clinical diseases and female reproductive problems. In addition to obtaining clinical history, additional diagnostic testing may be required, including hematological assessments. This article describes common blood collection methods, including venipuncture sites, volume of blood that can be safely collected, and handling of the blood. Hematological parameters for normal ferrets are provided along with a description of the morphology of ferret leukocytes to assist in performing a differential count.

Pet rabbits are presented to veterinary clinics for routine care and treatment of clinical diseases. In addition to obtaining clinical history and exam findings, diagnostic testing may be required, including hematological assessments. This article describes common blood collection methods, including venipuncture sites, volume of blood that can be safely collected, and handling of the blood. Hematological parameters for normal rabbits are provided for comparison with in-house or commercial test results. A description of the morphology of rabbit leukocytes is provided to assist in performing a differential count. Differential diagnoses are provided for abnormal values identified in the hemogram.

Hamsters, gerbils, rats, and mice are presented to veterinary clinics and hospitals for prophylactic care and treatment of clinical signs of disease. Physical examination, history, and husbandry practice information can be supplemented greatly by assessment of hematologic parameters. As a resource for veterinarians and their technicians, this article describes the methods for collection of blood, identification of blood cells, and interpretation of the hemogram in mice, rats, gerbils, and hamsters.

Pet guinea pigs are presented to veterinary clinics for routine care and treatment of clinical diseases. In addition to obtaining clinical history, diagnostic testing may be required, including hematological assessments. This

require additional equipment, may be inexpensive, and provide useful information in guiding treatment options. Challenges involving hematology may include handling and restraint, venipuncture, evaluation, and interpretation. In this article, strategies for these challenges are discussed for teleost (bony fish) and elasmobranch (cartilaginous fish) fish types.

Historically, reference intervals (RI) have come from many sources and been generated by several methods and sample sizes. As RI generation has matured in human laboratory medicine, important guidelines have been adopted in veterinary medicine. Although meeting the goals of these guidelines may be difficult, especially with avian and exotic species, sets of 20 to 40 samples can be used with proper statistical calculations, and other viable alternatives have been examined. The adoption and knowledge of these different methods are important to make a positive move forward in RI generation for special species.

Evaluation of hemic cell morphology in stained blood film may be the most important part of the hematologic evaluation of exotic animals. The blood film provides important information regarding red blood cell abnormalities, such as changes in cell shape and color, presence of inclusions, and, in the case of lower vertebrates, changes in the position of the cell nucleus. Stained blood film also provides information about changes in leukocyte numbers and morphology, and shows important hemic features of mammalian platelets and the thrombocytes of lower vertebrates. The blood film is needed in the detection and identification of blood parasites.

Special Articles

The need to rapidly diagnose disease in avian/exotic animal patients has led to the increased use of on-site diagnostic testing by veterinarians treating these animals. This article explores the use of on-site veterinary diagnostic testing: advantages and disadvantages of such testing; tests that are performed; type of equipment available; and the need for quality control.

The decision to purchase an in-office hematology instrument is typically based on the desire to have immediate access to complete blood count (CBC) data for disease diagnosis and follow-up and perhaps add to the financial bottom line of your practice. The decision regarding which in-office hematology instrument to purchase requires comparison of available instruments, how they function and knowledge of their strengths and limitations, what analytes they report, their ease of use, and their initial and continued costs. Other considerations include instrument space requirements, ability to interact with your existing data management system, the methods used by analyzers, and data accuracy.

VETERINARY CLINICS OF NORTH AMERICA: EXOTIC ANIMAL PRACTICE

RELATED INTEREST

Veterinary Clinics of North America: Small Animal Practice,
November 2012 (Vol. 42, No. 6)
Hematology
Joanne B. Messick, *Editor*

THE CLINICS ARE NOW AVAILABLE ONLINE!
Access your subscription at:
www.theclinics.com

VETERINARY CLINICS OF
NORTH AMERICA: EXOTIC
ANIMAL PRACTICE

FORTHCOMING ISSUES

May 2015
Wellness and Environmental Enrichment
Agnes E. Rupley, Editor

September 2015
Endoscopy
Stephen J. Divers and Jill M. Pecoros,
Editors

January 2016
Soft Tissue Surgery
Kurt Sladky and Christoph Mans,
Editors

RECENT ISSUES

September 2014
Nutrition
2014 Mayer Editor

May 2014
Gastroenterology
Tracey K. Ritzman, Editor

January 2014
Topics in Endocrinology
Anthony A. Pilny, Editor

RELATED INTEREST

Veterinary Clinics of North America: Small Animal Practice
November 2013 (Vol. 43, No. 6)
Hematology
Joanne B. Messick, Editor

Preface

Exotic Animal Hematology

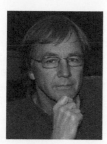

Terry W. Campbell, MS, DVM, PhD
Editor

In the early 1980s while I was working on my residency and toward a PhD in Veterinary Clinical Pathology at Kansas State University, I took up an interest in avian hematology. In those days, there was very little information on the subject. The only reference that I had to work with was the *Atlas of Avian Hematology* by AJ Lucas and C Jamroz, published in 1961 by the US Department of Agriculture (Monograph 25; Washington, DC: US Government Printing Office). I remember sitting down at the microscope focusing on the Wright's stained blood cells from a parrot and immediately feeling lost. All the hemic cells were nucleated! I was not used to that because my training in mammalian hematology involved anucleated erythrocytes and platelets. I nearly gave up. Yet, I pressed on with the help of my reference book and its beautifully hand-drawn images of cells found in the blood of domestic fowl. Today, of course, there are other references available to the veterinary practitioner, including this one, that contain photomicrographic images of the hemic cells of various exotic animal species. In my practice, I still find that examination of the hemic cytology and the hemogram of all exotic animal species can provide important diagnostic clues to the nature of my patient's illness.

This issue of *Veterinary Clinics of North America: Exotic Animal Practice* is devoted to the hematology of exotic animals with an emphasis on pet species. The authors lend their experiences and talents to guide the reader in the assessment of hemic cytology and the interpretation of hematologic data. The issue begins with the hematology of exotic mammalian species, which most veterinarians dealing with domestic mammals will likely find familiar. Hematology of mammals is followed by the nonmammalian articles, beginning with avian hematology. The reader will find similarities in the hematology of reptiles and fish to that of avian hematology. Meaningful reference values have been a challenge to obtain in the lower vertebrates; that is to say, animals with nucleated erythrocytes and thrombocytes, which is addressed next in this issue. When only a single drop of blood can be obtained from the exotic animal patient, the value of examination of the blood film is addressed in the final article.

Vet Clin Exot Anim 18 (2015) xi–xii
http://dx.doi.org/10.1016/j.cvex.2014.09.013
1094-9194/15/$ – see front matter © 2015 Elsevier Inc. All rights reserved.

I wish to express my sincere appreciation for the extra effort that each of my contributors has given to the development of this issue. Without their help, I and the publishing staff would not have been able to accomplish this publication within the timeframe and with the exceptional results. Working with these individuals has taught me the meaning of being colleagues.

Terry W. Campbell, MS, DVM, PhD
Department of Clinical Sciences
College of Veterinary Medicine and
Biomedical Sciences
Colorado State University
300 West Drake Road
Fort Collins, CO 80523, USA

E-mail address:
terry.campbell@colostate.edu

Hematology of the Domestic Ferret (*Mustela putorius furo*)

Stephen A. Smith, MS, DVM, PhD[a],*,
Kurt Zimmerman, DVM, PhD, DACVP[a],
David M. Moore, MS, DVM, DACLAM[b]

KEYWORDS

- Ferret • Blood collection • Hematology • Hemogram • White blood cells

KEY POINTS

- Today, the ferret is an important laboratory animal used in biomedical research as a model for a number of important human clinical syndromes and disease processes, such as Reye syndrome, *Helicobacter* gastritis, and antiemetic drug screening.
- Pet ferrets are presented to veterinary clinics for routine care and treatment of clinical diseases and female reproductive problems.
- In addition to obtaining clinical history, additional diagnostic testing may be required, including hematological assessments. This article describes common blood collection methods, including venipuncture sites, volume of blood that can be safely collected, and handling of the blood.

The domestic ferret (*Mustela putorius furo*) belongs to the family Mustelidae in the order Carnivora. They have been domesticated for more than a thousand years and were historically used for hunting of animals that lived in burrows. Today, the ferret is an important laboratory animal used in biomedical research as a model for a number of important human clinical syndromes and disease processes, such as Reye syndrome, *Helicobacter* gastritis, and antiemetic drug screening. There are 2 basic color types, the fitch and albino, but there are more than 30 recognized color combinations. Ferrets may live up to 12 years, but more commonly have a life span of 5 to 8 years. Males (hobs) may weigh 1 to 2 kg, and the smaller females (jills) may weigh 500 to 900 g.

[a] Department of Biomedical Sciences and Pathobiology, Virginia-Maryland Regional College of Veterinary Medicine, Virginia Tech, 245 Duck Pond Drive, Blacksburg, VA 24061, USA; [b] North End Center, Virginia Tech, 300 Turner Street Northwest, Suite 4120, Blacksburg, VA 24061, USA
* Corresponding author.
E-mail address: stsmith7@vt.edu

Vet Clin Exot Anim 18 (2015) 1–8
http://dx.doi.org/10.1016/j.cvex.2014.09.005
1094-9194/15/$ – see front matter © 2015 Elsevier Inc. All rights reserved.

In 2012, approximately 748,000 ferrets were maintained as pets in approximately 334,000 households in the United States.[1] As a resource for veterinarians and their technicians, this article describes the methods for collection of blood and identification of blood cells in ferrets.

METHODOLOGY FOR BLOOD COLLECTION
Restraint

Proper techniques for handling and restraint of ferrets have been described in a number of publications.[2–5] A brief description of standard handling and restraint methods for ferrets is provided in the following sections.

Manual restraint
Specific manual restraint techniques are described in the section on venipuncture techniques.

Chemical restraint
Doses of anesthetics and tranquilizers used in ferrets are provided in other publications.[6,7] In general, anesthesia is not required for most blood collection procedures, and based on the clinical status of the patient at the time of presentation, the clinician should determine whether an animal should or should not be anesthetized. For sedation, midazolam (midazolam 0.25–1.0 mg/kg intramuscularly) may be used, or general anesthesia, using isoflurane or sevoflurane, can be used if the handler or phlebotomist is relatively inexperienced. Isoflurane may adversely affect the results of blood parameters in ferrets, and this should be considered when interpreting the results.[8,9] Total red cell, white cell, and platelet numbers can be significantly lower in anesthetized ferrets.[9,10]

Blood Collection Sites: Location and Preparation, and Venipuncture Techniques

Blood collection techniques in a ferret are comparable to those in the cat. Common sites used for blood collection are the lateral saphenous vein, the cephalic vein, the jugular vein, dorsal metatarsal vein, and the cranial vena cava.[2,11–15] Less common sites, not recommended in a private practice setting, are the caudal artery of the tail, and the orbital sinus. Depending on the vessel selected, a 22-gauge to 30-gauge needle should be used. For smaller veins, a 1-mL syringe should be used to prevent collapse of the vessel during aspiration of the blood sample.

The jugular vein is the most accessible site for the collection of blood in the domestic ferret. A variety of restraint techniques may be used. The ferret may be placed in dorsal or lateral recumbency with the head extended and the front legs pulled/restrained in a caudal direction. The fur should be clipped over the venipuncture site, and the area swabbed with an appropriate disinfectant solution. The ferret jugular vein, as compared with that in the cat, runs in a more lateral position. A 22-gauge to 25-gauge needle is inserted into the vein in a cranial direction, and the blood aspirated into the syringe. After the needle is withdrawn, firm pressure should be applied to prevent hematoma formation. A second method involves placing the animal in sternal recumbency, pulling the front legs downward over the edge of the examination table, and flexing the head in a caudal direction. A third method involves having the animal held by the scruff of the neck by one individual, suspended perpendicular to the floor or examination table, while the phlebotomist performs the venipuncture. In this technique, the needle and syringe are parallel to the floor, and the needle is inserted perpendicular to the ferret. A fourth method involves wrapping the animal securely in a towel, with the head and neck exposed.

The cranial vena cava[16] also can be used to obtain blood; however, the ferret should be sedated to reduce the risk of laceration of the vessel by the needle (should the animal move), resulting in significant internal hemorrhage. In the unanesthetized ferret, 2 handlers should provide restraint of the animal. The animal is placed in dorsal recumbency on the examination table, one individual restraining and stabilizing the head, and the other individual restraining the lower body and drawing the front legs in a caudal direction. The fur should be clipped over the venipuncture site, and the area swabbed with an appropriate disinfectant solution. The needle is inserted in the right thoracic notch (the animal's right side), the space between the manubrium and the first rib. A 25-gauge to 27-gauge 0.5-inch needle, held at a 30° angle with respect to the plane of the body, is inserted in a caudolateral direction, "aiming" it toward the left hip. As the needle is inserted, the phlebotomist should draw back on the plunger of the syringe to create negative pressure. Once blood is seen to flow into the needle hub or syringe, the phlebotomist will stop insertion of the needle, and stabilize the needle and syringe to complete the collection of the sample. After the needle is withdrawn, pressure should be applied to the site, but this will only prevent flow of blood from the puncture in the skin, but not stop any flow that might occur within the thoracic cavity.

The lateral saphenous may be used for collecting small amounts of blood for packed cell volume (PCV) or complete blood count. As with the vena cava collection, 2 persons should manually restrain the unanesthetized ferret for blood collection by the phlebotomist. The fur over the venipuncture site, on the lateral aspect below the stifle, should be clipped, and the area swabbed with an appropriate disinfectant solution. One individual restrains the animal's upper body, and the second individual restrains the lower body, and restrains the leg and applies pressure over the vessel at a point above the stifle. Alternatively, a Penrose drain may be used as a tourniquet. A 25-gauge to 27-gauge needle on a 0.5-mL to 1.0-mL syringe is inserted in a proximal direction in the vessel, with the phlebotomist applying slow, gentle aspiration to prevent the vein from collapsing. After the needle is withdrawn, firm pressure should be applied to prevent hematoma formation.

The procedure for cephalic vein venipuncture and blood collection is similar to that in cats. However, because this vein is ideal for intravenous catheter placement, it should perhaps be preserved by selecting an alternate venipuncture site. Manual restraint can be accomplished by wrapping the animal in a towel, with the limb exposed. The animal also can be restrained by the scruff of the neck, and the limb extended, with digital pressure or a tourniquet applied proximal to the venipuncture site.

By outward appearance, blood collection via the caudal tail artery is painful or distressing to the animal. Additionally, hematological parameters can vary greatly when blood is collected by this method.[2] One individual restrains the animal in dorsal recumbency. The phlebotomist, using a 20-gauge to 21-gauge needle on a 1-mL to 3-mL syringe, inserts the needle into the groove on the midline of the ventral surface of the tail, beginning about 1 to 2 inches (2–5 cm) from the base of the tail, and inserting the needle at a 45° angle in a proximal direction. Because of the arterial pressure, the arteriopuncture site should be held off for 3 minutes or longer to ensure adequate hemostasis, and to prevent hematoma formation.

Volume Collected

The estimated whole blood volume, based on body weight, and the recommended maximum safe blood volume that should be considered, are provided in **Table 1**. It would be prudent to collect a smaller volume of blood (0.5% of body weight) from geriatric, anemic, hypoproteinemic, or otherwise clinically ill patients.

Table 1
Determining maximum safe blood sample volumes in ferrets based on body weight

Body Weight (kg)	Whole Blood Volume (mL) (5%–6% of Body Weight)	Draw No More than 7.5%–10% of WBV (Safe Volume to Collect - mL)
0.5	25–30	1.88–3
0.75	37.5–45	2.8–4.5
1.0	50–60	3.75–6
1.25	62.5–75	4.7–7.5
1.50	75–90	5.6–9
1.75	87.5–105	6.6–10.5
2.0	100–120	7.5–12

Abbreviation: WBV, whole blood volume.

MORPHOLOGY AND NUMBERS OF PERIPHERAL BLOOD CELLS

Anesthesia, sex, age, reproductive cycle, circadian rhythm, restraint, stress, and the site of blood sampling can affect hemogram results. A generalized reference range for normal hematological values reported for the domestic ferret is listed in **Table 2**.[17–20] More complete hematologic reference intervals or individual-specific values may be found scattered throughout the ferret literature.[21–26]

Most values are similar to values reported for other domestic carnivores; however, the hematocrit, hemoglobin, and total erythrocyte and reticulocyte counts in ferrets are generally higher than in the dog or cat.[27] Additionally, ferrets have no detectable blood groups and therefore no naturally occurring antibodies against unmatched erythrocyte antigens. Therefore, repeated transfusions without the development of antibodies are possible in the ferret.[27]

Table 2
Referenced ranges of normal hematological parameters in the ferret (*Mustela putorius furo*)

Parameter	Adult Male	Adult Female	Age 2–3 mo
RBC ($\times 10^6$/μL)	6.5–13.2	6.7–9.34	4.8–7.8
PCV (%)	33.6–49.8	35.6–55	27.0–38.5
Hgb (g/dL)	12.0–18.2	12.9–17.4	9.6–13.8
MCV (fL)	44.1–52.5	44.4–53.7	47.8–57.6
MCH (pg)	16.5–19.7	16.4–19.4	17.5–22.8
MCHC (%)	33.7–42.2	33.2–35.3	34.7–37.0
Platelets ($\times 10^3$/μL)	297–730	310–910	—
WBC ($\times 10^3$/μL)	4.4–15.4	2.5–18.2	5.3–12.6
Neutrophils (%)	24–76	43–78	46.1–76.6
Lymphocytes (%)	12–66.6	12–67	42.2–68.2
Eosinophils (%)	0–8.5	0–8.5	2.1–6.9
Basophils (%)	0–3	0–2.9	0–1.3
Monocytes (%)	0–8.2	1–6.3	0.7–4.7

Abbreviations: Hgb, hemoglobin; MCH, mean corpuscular hemoglobin; MCHC, mean corpuscular hemoglobin concentration; MCV, mean corpuscular volume; PCV, packed cell volume; RBC, red blood cell; WBC, white blood cell.
Data from Refs.[17–20]

Erythrocytes (Red Blood Cell)

The mean red blood cell (RBC) diameter for ferrets is reported to be 5.94 μm (range of 4.6–7.7 μm) in males and 6.32 μm (range of 4.6–7.7 μm) in females.[19,27–29] The hematocrit of ferrets ranges between 30% and 61%, but usually averages between 40% and 50% for adult ferrets and between 32% and 39% for juvenile ferrets. The mean percentage of reticulocytes is reported to be 4% (range of 1%–12%) in male ferrets and 5.3% (range of 2%–14%) in female ferrets.[19] Low numbers of Howell-Jolly bodies have been reported in a small percentage of both male and female ferrets. Other red blood cell values are listed in **Table 2**.[19,29]

Jills are induced ovulators, and individuals that do not breed during estrus may exhibit prolonged estrus throughout the breeding season. After a month of prolonged estrus, high levels of estrogen in the bloodstream may cause bone marrow suppression with leucopenia, thrombocytopenia, and aplastic anemia. A decrease in PCV and total RBC numbers in jills is consistent with prolonged estrus. Jills with PCV values higher than 25% generally have a good prognosis, and ovariohysterectomy will quickly remove high circulating estrogen levels with a return to normal erythrocyte production in the bone marrow. Alternatively, hormone treatments such as proligestone, human chorionic gonadotrophin, or gonadotrophin-releasing hormone injections can be used to induce ovulation, resulting in decreased circulating estrogen levels. However, it might take up to 4 months for the anemia to fully resolve. PCV values between 15% and 25% in jills present a guarded prognosis, and supportive care, such as fluid replacement and blood transfusion, may be indicated before any surgery is attempted. As described previously, administration of hormone injections also can be considered. The prognosis for jills with a PCV lower than 15% is poor, and may require blood transfusions over several months.

A polychromatophil, an immature RBC that has lost its nucleus, appears bluer than a mature RBC (when Wright's stain is used), and it is usually larger than a mature RBC. Polychromatophilia is suggestive of an increased production of erythrocytes by the bone marrow (erythroid hyperplasia) in response to anemia. The presence of clinical signs of prolonged estrus with anemia can be confirmed with the presence of increased numbers of polychromatophils. A representative polychromatophil is shown in **Fig. 1**B.

Thrombocytes (Platelets)

The mean platelet diameter for male and female ferrets is reported to be 1.7 μm (range of 1.5–2.3 μm).[19,28] The mean number of circulating platelets reported in ferrets varies significantly between studies.[17,30] As noted previously, a jill with prolonged estrus may have a low platelet count. Referenced values for platelet counts in normal ferrets is provided in **Table 2**.

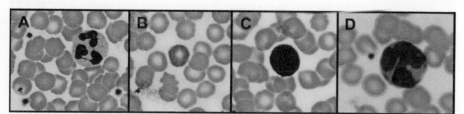

Fig. 1. Representative ferret blood cells. (A) Neutrophil, RBCs, and platelets. (B) Polychromatophil and RBCs. (C) Lymphocyte and RBCs. (D) Monocyte and RBCs. (Wright-Giemsa stain, original magnification 1000×).

Leukocytes (White Blood Cells)

Neutrophils are the predominant leukocyte observed in ferret blood, followed by lymphocytes, eosinophils and monocytes, and finally basophils. The ranges of total white blood cell (WBC) numbers and the WBC cell types observed in a standard differential count are provided in **Table 2**.

Neutrophils

The ferret neutrophil has a segmented nucleus, and its pale blue cytoplasm contains polychromatic granules. Comparative values of neutrophils observed in differential counts in normal ferrets, by age and sex, are provided in **Table 2**. A typical neutrophil is illustrated in **Fig. 1A**.

Lymphocytes

Ferret lymphocytes have a reported mean diameter of 7.7 μm (range of 6.2–9.2 μm) in males and 8.7 μm (range of 7.7–10.0 μm) in females.[19] Comparative values of lymphocytes observed in differential counts in normal ferrets, by age and sex, are provided in **Table 2**. A typical lymphocyte is illustrated in **Fig. 1C**.

Eosinophils

Eosinophils may have a 1-lobed or 2-lobed nucleus, and the cytoplasm is filled with numerous round red granules. Eosinophils have a mean diameter of 12.7 μm in males and 12.6 μm in females.[19,29] Comparative values of eosinophils observed in differential counts in normal ferrets, by age and sex, are provided in **Table 2**.

Basophils

Basophils have a segmented nucleus with a reported mean diameter of 13.5 μm in males and 13.8 μm in females.[19] Comparative values of basophils observed in differential counts in normal ferrets, by age and sex, are provided in **Table 2**.

Monocytes

Monocytes have a reported diameter between 12 and 18 μm. Comparative values of monocytes observed in differential counts in normal ferrets, by age and sex, are provided in **Table 2**. A typical lymphocyte is illustrated in **Fig. 1D**.

REFERENCES

1. American Veterinary Medical Association. 2012 U.S. pet ownership & demographic sourcebook. Schaumberg (IL): AVMA; 2012.
2. Joslin JO. Blood collection techniques in exotic small mammals. J EXOT PET MED 2009;18(2):117–39.
3. Hrapkiewicz K, Colby L, Denison P. Clinical laboratory animal medicine: an introduction. 4th edition. Ames (IA): Wiley Blackwell; 2013. p. 298–307.
4. Fox JG. Housing and management. In: Fox JG, editor. Biology and diseases of the ferret. 2nd edition. Baltimore (MD): Williams & Wilkins; 1998. p. 179–80.
5. Ballard B, Rockett J. Restraint and handling for veterinary technicians and assistants. Clifton Park (NY): Delmar; 2009. p. 70–2.
6. Drexel University. A compendium of drugs used for laboratory animal anesthesia, analgesia, tranquilization and restraint. Philadelphia: Drexel University IACUC; 2007.

7. Marini RP, Fox JG. Anesthesia, surgery, and biomethodology. In: Fox JG, editor. Biology and diseases of the ferret. 2nd edition. Baltimore: Williams & Wilkins; 1998. p. 464–72.
8. Ness RD. Clinical pathology and sample collection of exotic small mammals. Vet Clin North Am Exot Anim Pract 1999;2:591–620.
9. Marini RP. Effect of isoflurane on hematologic variables in ferrets. Am J Vet Res 1994;55:1479–83.
10. Marini R, Callahan R, Jackson L. Distribution of technetium 99m-labeled red blood cells during isoflurane anesthesia in ferrets. Am J Vet Res 1997;58:781–5.
11. Bleakley SP. Simple technique for bleeding ferrets (Mustela putorius furo). Lab Anim 1980;14:59–60.
12. Brown S. Clinical techniques in domestic ferrets. Seminar Avian Exotic Pet Med 1997;6:75–85.
13. Capello V. Application of the cranial vena cava venipuncture technique to small exotic mammals. Exot DVM 2006:8.3, Zoological Education Network.
14. Dyer SM, Cervasio EL. An overview of restraint and blood collection techniques in exotic pet practice. Vet Clin North Am Exot Anim Pract 2008;11:423–43.
15. Otto G, Rosenblad WD, Fox JG. Practical venipuncture techniques for the ferret. Lab Anim 1993;27:26–9.
16. Brown C. Blood collection from the cranial vena cava of the ferret. Lab Anim (NY) 2006;35(9):23–4.
17. Besch-Williford CL. Biology and medicine of the ferret. Vet Clin North Am Small Anim Pract 1987;17:1155–83.
18. Fox JG, Marini R. Diseases of the endocrine system. In: Fox JG, editor. Biology and diseases of the ferret. Baltimore (MD): Williams & Wilkins; 1998. p. 291–305.
19. Thornton PC. The ferret Mustela putorius furo, as a new species in toxicology. Lab Anim 1979;13:119–24.
20. Zimmerman KL, Moore MM, Smith SA. Hematology of the ferret. In: Weiss DJ, Wardrop KJ, editors. Schalm's veterinary hematology. Ames (IA): Wiley-Blackwell; 2010. p. 904–9.
21. Carpenter JW, Hill EF. Hematological values for the Siberian ferret. J Zoo Anim Med 1979;10:126–8.
22. Fox JG. Serum chemistry and hematology reference values in the ferret. Lab Anim Sci 1986;36:22–8.
23. Hoover JP, Baldwin CA. Changes in physiologic and clinicopathologic values in domestic ferrets from 12–47 weeks of age. Companion Anim Pract 1988;2: 40–4.
24. Lee EJ. Haematological and serum chemistry profiles of ferrets (Mustela putorius furo). Lab Anim 1982;16:133–7.
25. Ohwada K, Katahira K. Reference values for organ weight, hematology and serum chemistry in the female ferret (Mustela putorius furo). Jikken Dobutsu 1993;42:135–42.
26. Zeissler R. Hematological and clinical biochemical parameters in ferrets under various physiological and pathological conditions. 1. Comparative studies of changes in the hemograms of pregnant, lactating and non-pregnant females. Z Versuchstierkd 1981;23:244–54.
27. Marini R, Otto G, Erdman S. Biology and diseases of the ferret. In: Fox JG, Anderson L, Lowe F, editors. Laboratory animal medicine. London: Academic Press; 2002. p. 483–517.
28. Hillyer EV, Quesenberry KE. Ferrets rabbits, and rodents: clinical medicine and surgery. Philadelphia: WB Saunders; 1997. p. 432.

29. Siperstein LJ. Ferret hematology and related disorders. Vet Clin North Am Exot Anim Pract 2008;11:535–50.
30. Kawasaki TA. Normal parameters and laboratory interpretation of disease states in the domestic ferret. Semin Avian Exotic Pet Med 1994;3:40–7.

Hematological Assessment in Pet Rabbits

Blood Sample Collection and Blood Cell Identification

David M. Moore, MS, DVM, DACLAM[a],*,
Kurt Zimmerman, DVM, PhD, DACVP[b], Stephen A. Smith, DVM, PhD[b]

KEYWORDS

- Rabbit • Blood collection • Hematology • Hemogram
- White blood cell count morphology • Differential count

KEY POINTS

- Part of the clinical care of pet rabbits is the assessment of overt and latent clinical conditions, and hematological assessments are an important part of the clinician's armamentarium.

The American Veterinary Medical Association (AVMA) has estimated that about 1.4 million households have pet rabbits, with a total of 3.2 million rabbits maintained as pets.[1] Because about two-thirds of pet owners consider their pets to be family members, it is important that Flopsy, Mopsy, and Cottontail receive the clinical care they need and deserve. Part of that clinical care is the assessment of overt and latent clinical conditions, and hematological assessments are an important part of the clinician's armamentarium. Because indoor-housed rabbits have a lifespan of 8 to 12 years (and outdoor-housed have a lifespan of about 4–8 years), visits to the veterinary clinic may add up over time. This article describes the methods for manual restraint, collection of blood, identification of blood cells, and interpretation of the hemogram in rabbits.

METHODOLOGY FOR BLOOD COLLECTION
Restraint

A rabbit presented for clinical evaluation may already be stressed from transport to the clinic, and from the sights, sounds, and smells in the clinic. Those stressors may

[a] Virginia Tech, 300 Turner Street Northwest, Suite 4120 (0497), Blacksburg, VA 24061, USA;
[b] Department of Biomedical Sciences and Pathobiology (0442), Virginia–Maryland Regional College of Veterinary Medicine, 245 Duck Pond Drive, Blacksburg, VA 24061, USA
* Corresponding author.
E-mail address: moored@vt.edu

Vet Clin Exot Anim 18 (2015) 9–19
http://dx.doi.org/10.1016/j.cvex.2014.09.003
1094-9194/15/$ – see front matter © 2015 Elsevier Inc. All rights reserved.

engage the flight response in the rabbit, and attempts to flee from the examination table may have disastrous consequences. To avoid injury to its spine, be sure to support the rabbit's hindquarters when picking it up to move it from 1 location to another.

Although manual restraint may be used for auscultation and palpation of the rabbit, potentially stressful procedures, such as blood collection, are best accomplished with additional restraint devices, to reduce the risk of injury to the patient and to the technician or veterinarian. A rabbit can scratch and slash handlers with the claws on its forefeet and hind feet, and struggling and twisting by an inadequately restrained rabbit may result in spine and spinal cord injury in the animal, with either paresis or permanent paralysis as the outcome. Most clinics have cloth cat restraint bags in multiple sizes, and an appropriately sized bag can be used to restrain a rabbit. Alternatively, a bath towel can be used to wrap up the rabbit, leaving its head exposed. The slight pressure that both of those exert on the rabbit's body provides a calming effect, and the rabbit is unlikely to struggle and injure its spine. Chemical restraint may also be used to facilitate blood collection; however, anesthesia may be contraindicated in an already debilitated patient. Drugs that can be used in sedation, tranquilization, and anesthesia of rabbits have been described in the published literature.[2,3]

Blood Collection Sites—Location and Preparation, and Venipuncture Techniques

The 2 primary vessels used for blood collection from a rabbit are the marginal ear vein, yielding small-to-moderate quantities of blood (depending on the experience and expertise of the phlebotomist), and the central auricular artery, from which a larger volume of blood can be collected. Other veins/sites that may be used include the lateral saphenous vein of the hind leg, the cephalic vein on the foreleg, and the jugular vein. Restraint required for those alternate sites may be stressful to the animal. Thus the 2 preferred methods are emphasized in this article.

Table 1 provides a comparison of the advantages and disadvantages of the common blood collection sites in rabbits. **Fig. 1** illustrates the location of the 2 preferred vessels for blood collection in the rabbit.

The central auricular artery and the marginal ear vein(s) are approached on the outer, haired surface of the pinna of either ear. The fur should be plucked over the intended venipuncture site. This is not distressful to the rabbit, and the minor local irritation stimulates vasodilation. The venipuncture site should be cleansed with a suitable disinfectant solution or alcohol, recognizing that this may result in vasoconstriction. Induction of vasodilation, and thus facilitation of blood collection, can be accomplished by several procedures, and technicians and veterinarians may select among the methods listed to accomplish that aim:

- Fill an examination glove with water. Tie it off; microwave it until its temperature is warm to the touch, but not scalding, and apply that to the rabbit's era for about a minute.
- Swab the skin over the proposed venipuncture site with oil of wintergreen and then collect blood 1 to 2 minutes after its application, taking care to rinse any residual oil off the ear after the blood has been collected.
- Administer acepromazine subcutaneously (0.5–1.0 mg/kg) about 15 to 20 minutes before blood collection (the time involved is perhaps not practical in a busy practice).
- Gently stroke (milk) the vessel with the thumb and forefinger from the base of the ear toward the tip of the ear.

Recommended needle sizes range from 22 to 25 gauge, selecting the smallest gauge needle required to minimize discomfort and tissue trauma. Standard needles

Table 1
Comparison of blood collection sites in the rabbit

Collection Site	Advantages	Disadvantages
Marginal ear vein	• Easily visualized • Easily accessible • Vessel is not mobile • Does not require sedation/anesthesia • Good for collecting small volumes of blood	• The vein is small and easily collapsed with rapid aspiration • May be too small in smaller breeds or young rabbits • Cannot collect a large volume of blood • May result in thrombosis and sloughing of skin over site • Hematoma formation and bruising can occur
Central auricular artery	• Easily visualized • Easily accessible • Vessel is not mobile • Does not require sedation/anesthesia • Rapid collection of larger volume of blood	• May require topical application of a local anesthetic to prevent arteriospasm • If damage is done to the artery, blood supply to the pinna will be compromised • Hematoma formation and bruising can occur
Lateral saphenous vein	• Easily visualized • Easily accessible	• Vein is mobile, requires stabilization • Vein may collapse during aspiration • Sedation desirable to prevent injury to limb
Cephalic vein	• Good for collecting small-to-moderate volumes of blood	• May not be easily visualized • Vein is mobile, requires stabilization • Sedation desirable to prevent injury to limb and visual stress to rabbit • Skin may be contaminated with exudates from upper respiratory tract (URT) infection—foreleg used in grooming • Shorter length in smaller breeds, hard to access
Jugular vein	• Good for collecting larger volumes of blood	• Not easily visualized in obese rabbits or females with large dewlaps • Sedation/anesthesia recommended • Short nosed/dwarf breeds and rabbits with URT infections may become dypsneic when the neck is extended back during restraint

or butterfly catheters may be used. The vacuum associated with a vacutainer tube may collapse the vessel; thus use of a syringe is recommended to control the rate of aspiration.

The lateral, as opposed to the medial, marginal ear vein is the more accessible of the 2 veins. One individual, using a thumb and forefinger, should apply pressure to the vein near the base of the ear. The needle is inserted into the vein, directing it toward the base of the ear. The skin and vessel wall are thin enough to visualize the needle within the vessel. The phlebotomist should slowly aspirate the blood, pausing briefly if the flow has stopped, or slowly rotating the needle and syringe on its axis in case the bevel of the needle has been closed off by the vessel wall. When the needle is withdrawn, the assistant/technician should apply gentle pressure over the venipuncture site with a cotton swab or sterile gauze pad for about 1 to 2 minutes to prevent hematoma formation.

When collecting blood from the central auricular artery (**Fig. 2**), the phlebotomist should apply digital pressure to the artery near the tip of the era, and insert the needle in a distal direction, toward the base of the ear. Given the higher pressure in the artery,

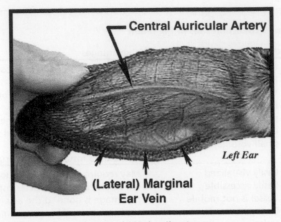

Fig. 1. Vessels of the rabbit ear used for blood collection.

gentle pressure should be applied over the venipuncture site for 2 to 4 minutes (or as needed) to prevent hematoma formation. A hematoma on the pinna may be irritating to the rabbit, causing head shaking and ear scratching, which can cause the hematoma to become even larger and more irritating.

Several publications are available that provide additional information on restraint and blood collection in rabbits.[4,5]

Volume Collected

Depending on the number and types of blood tests (eg, complete blood cell count [CBC], differential, and/or clinical chemistry) and the size and strain of rabbit, 0.5 to 10 mL of blood can be withdrawn using the methods described previously. The recommended maximum safe volume of blood that can be collected is 7.7 mL/kg of body weight.[6]

Handling of the Blood Sample

A drop of fresh blood, without anticoagulant, can be placed on a clean glass microscope slide for preparation of a peripheral blood smear for examination for the differential count of leukocytes, and for assessing erythrocyte abnormalities. Fresh blood can be drawn into heparinized microhematocrit tubes for determination of the packed cell volume (hematocrit).

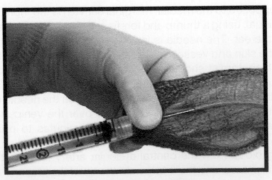

Fig. 2. Blood collection from the central auricular artery.

If additional tests are to be performed (eg, total/absolute white cell count or clinical chemistry testing), the blood should be placed in a vacutainer tube containing anticoagulant (a purple top tube containing Ethylenediaminetetraacetic acid [EDTA]). To minimize the risk of hemolysis of red blood cells, which would adversely affect test results, the following steps should be taken:

- Remove the rubber stopper from the vacutainer.
- Remove the needle from the syringe containing the blood.
- Slowly dispense the blood down an inside wall of the tube.
- Gently agitate the tube to mix the blood with the anticoagulant.

Samples may be stored at 4°C prior to testing, and timely processing (eg, within 1 hour after collection) is preferable. Overnight shipment to outside laboratories and testing within 48 to 72 hours should yield analytically acceptable results.[7]

MORPHOLOGY AND NUMBERS OF PERIPHERAL BLOOD CELLS
Erythrocytes

The rabbit erythrocyte is a biconcave disc with an average diameter of 6.7 to 6.9 μm,[8] and an average thickness of 2.15 to 2.4 μm.[9,10] The average lifespan of an erythrocyte ranges from 45 to 70 days.[6] There can be marked variability in the size of erythrocytes, referred to as anisocytosis, with some cells being one-fourth the diameter of normal cells.[11]

Polychromasia, a variation in staining of erythrocytes with Wright's stain, associated with the presence of young erythrocytes, those cells having a diffuse blue color, was observed in 1% to 2% of erythrocytes.[9] Young rabbits, 1 to 2 months of age, were found to have reticulocyte counts of 3% to 11%; adult males were found to have reticulocyte counts of 1.5% to 2.5%; and adult females were found to have reticulocyte counts of 2.5% to 3.5%.[10,11] Higher reticulocyte counts may be found after repeated blood collections, and are associated with regenerative anemia.[12,13]

Comparative values of erythrocyte parameters in rabbits are provided in **Tables 2** and **3**. Male rabbits have slightly higher numbers of erythrocytes and slightly higher hemoglobin concentrations compared with females.[6] Compared with adults, newborn rabbits have lower erythrocyte counts; however, their mean corpuscular volume (MCV) and mean corpuscular hemoglobin (MCH) values are higher than those in adults.

Thrombocytes (Platelets)

Comparative values of thrombocyte numbers are provided in **Table 2**. Thrombocytes may be observed singly or in groups in stained blood smears. They may be oblong, oval, or rounded, and they may be from 1 μm to 3 μm in diameter. When stained with Wright's stain, they appear to have a violet-hued center, with a pale blue to colorloos periphery.[14] It was observed that in acute infectious processes, there is a decrease in thrombocyte counts and an increase in nucleated red blood cell (RBC) counts.[15]

Leukocytes (White Blood Cells)

The ranges of total white blood cell (WBC) numbers and the WBC types observed in a standard differential count are provided in **Tables 2** and **3**. The WBC count in rabbits may vary dramatically as a result of circadian rhythms (diurnal fluctuations and variation within a month), nutritional status and dietary differences, and differences in age, gender, and breed.[6] Total leukocyte counts are lowest in the late afternoon and evening.[16]

Table 2
Referenced ranges of normal hematological parameters in the New Zealand white rabbit (*oryctolagus cuniculus*)

	Adult Male	Adult Female	Age 1 to 3 mo
RBC ($\times 10^6$/μL)	5.46–7.94	5.11–6.51	5.15–6.48
PCV (%)	33–50	31.0–48.6	38.1–44.1
Hgb (g/dL)	10.4–17.4	9.8–15.8	10.7–13.9
MCV (fL)	58.5–66.5	57.8–65.4	66.2–80.3
MCH (pg)	18.7–22.7	17.1–23.5	19.5–22.7
MCHC (%)	33–50	28.7–35.7	24.2–32.6
Platelets ($\times 10^3$/μL)	304–656	270–630	—
WBC ($\times 10^3$/μL)	5.5–12.5	5.2–10.6	4.1–9.79
Neutrophils (%)	38–54	36.4–50.4	18.8–46.4
Lymphocytes (%)	28–50	31.5–52.1	44.6–77.8
Eosinophils (%)	0.5–3.5	0.8–3.2	0–2.4
Basophils (%)	2.5–7.5	2.4–6.2	0.1–4.5
Monocytes (%)	4–12	6.6–13.4	0–13.1

Data from Refs.[6,8,11]

Neutrophils

The rabbit neutrophil, also referred to as a heterophil, is the second most common WBC seen in peripheral blood smears. The rabbit neutrophil contains small acidophilic granules and varying numbers of large red granules, leading some to call it a pseudoeosinophil.[11] The smaller pink granules outnumber the larger red granules by 80% to 90%.[17] The rabbit neutrophil is about 10 μm to 15 μm in diameter; its polymorphic nucleus stains light purple, and the nucleus is surrounded by a diffusely pink cytoplasm.[11] A typical rabbit neutrophil is illustrated in **Fig. 3**.

Table 3
Referenced ranges of normal hematological parameters in 3 additional rabbit species

	Dutch Belted (*Lepus europaeus*)	Eastern Cottontail (*Sylvilagus floridianus*)	Jackrabbit (*Lepus californicus*)
RBC ($\times 10^6$/μL)	4.8–6.3	4.2	6.59–8.56
PCV (%)	34.8–48.9	18–49	42–53
Hgb (g/dL)	12.2–16.3	—	13.7–17.5
MCV (fL)	62.7–88.1	—	57.6–70.0
MCH (pg)	22.0–29.4	—	18–23.1
MCHC (%)	28.5–38.1	—	28.8–36.8
Platelets ($\times 10^3$/μL)	126–490	—	170–798
WBC ($\times 10^3$/μL)	6–13	—	2.2–14.7
Neutrophils (%)	30–50	0.5–61.5	13.0–81.5
Lymphocytes (%)	28.5–52.5	22–93	25–83
Eosinophils (%)	0.5–5.0	0.0–9.5	0–8
Basophils (%)	2–8	0.0–6.5	0.0–1.5
Monocytes (%)	2–16	0–5	2–10

Data from Refs.[6,8,11,23–25]

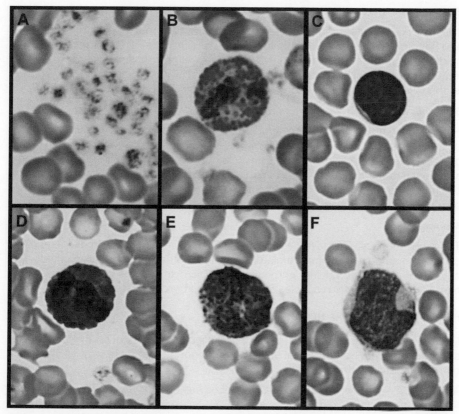

Fig. 3. Representative rabbit blood cells. (A) RBCs and platelets. (B) Heterophil, platelets, and RBCs. (C) Lymphocyte and RBCs. (D) Eosinophil and RBCs. (E) Basophil and RBCs. (F) Monocyte and RBCs. (Wright-Giemsa stain; 1000x).

The number of circulating neutrophils is lower in the early morning and highest in the late afternoon and evening.[16]

A rare homozygous genetic condition, the Pelger-Huet anomaly, has been observed in rabbits, and is characterized by severe skeletal deformities and higher mortality.[6] In this condition, neutrophils and monocytes are observed as having round-to-oval nuclei, without the typical segmentation. However, the presence of a few such cells in a blood smear from an otherwise normal rabbit are not indicative of the genetic condition.[14]

Lymphocytes

The lymphocyte is the most common WBC cell type observed in peripheral blood smears. The rabbit lymphocyte may be seen in both small and large forms, with the former about the size of an RBC, and the latter as large as a neutrophil.[14] The nucleus of the rabbit lymphocyte is condensed and round, and surrounded by a narrow band of blue-staining cytoplasm, which, in larger lymphocytes, may contain azurophilic granules.[18] The number of circulating lymphocytes is higher in the early morning, and lowest in the late afternoon and evening.[16] A typical rabbit lymphocyte is illustrated in **Fig. 3**.

Eosinophils

The rabbit eosinophil is slightly larger than a neutrophil (about 12–16 μm in diameter), and has a bilobed or horseshoe-shaped nucleus. Within the cytoplasm are numerous acidophilic granules that are about 3 to 4 times larger than those in neutrophils, which may occupy much of the space in the cytoplasm.[14,17] A low or absent eosinophil count is observed in healthy rabbits.[16] A typical rabbit eosinophil is illustrated in **Fig. 3**.

Basophils

Rabbits, in contrast to most other species, have small-to-moderate numbers of basophils in the peripheral circulation, in some instances constituting up to 30% of WBCs in differential counts in clinically normal animals.[17] The rabbit basophil is about the same size as the rabbit neutrophil. The basophil nucleus stains light purple, and the cytoplasm contains purple-to-black metachromic granules, which may sometimes obscure the nucleus.[14,17,18] A typical rabbit basophil is illustrated in **Fig. 3**.

Monocytes

The rabbit monocyte is the largest of the WBCs (around 15–18 μm in diameter). This cell has an amoeboid-shaped nucleus (lobulated, horseshoe, or bean-shaped), with diffuse, lightly stained nuclear chromatin.[11,18] The cytoplasm is blue in color, and it may occasionally contain vacuoles.[18] A typical rabbit lymphocyte is illustrated in **Fig. 3**.

INTERPRETATION OF THE HEMOGRAM

Differences in hematological values were assessed in 3 breeds of rabbits, and the results are provided; however, that same author reported that there was no significant difference between the breeds[19]:

Chinchilla—highest value for WBC, lymphocytes, monocytes, RBC, hemoglobon (Hb), packed cell volume (PCV) and MCV

New Zealand white—highest value for mean corpuscular hemoglobin concentration (MCHC) and MCH

Dutch—highest values in neutrophils, eosinophils, basophils, and platelets

Rabbits presenting with an infectious disease do not typically have a higher WBC count, but rather have a shift from lymphocyte-predominant to neutrophil-predominant differential counts. Sometimes rabbits with acute infections may have a normal differential count, but a decrease in total WBC count.[17] Leukemias are infrequently reported in rabbits, usually presented as lymphoblastic leukemia.[20] In cases of septicemia and in overwhelming bacterial infections, leucopenia with a degenerative left shift will be observed.

Rabbits transported at 28°C (82.4°F) for 1 to 3 hours were found to have elevated PCV, lymphocytopenia, and leukocytosis.[21] Cold stress has been shown to cause an increase in RBC numbers.[16] Clinicians should consider and note environmental temperatures associated with transport of rabbits to the clinic when conducting hematological examinations.

In an experimental study in rabbits of hepatic coccidiosis (caused by *Eimeria stiedai*), hematological findings 7 days after infection included anemia, leukocytosis, neutrophilia, and monocytosis.[22]

Erythrocytes

Low hematocrit/packed cell volume less than 30%
- Regenerative anemia (indicated by polychromasia, nucleated RBCs, and Howell-Jolly bodies [inclusions of nuclear chromatin remnants])[8]

- Varying degrees of anemia (present with chronic infectious conditions [eg, pasteurellosis], with associated abcessation of skin or internal organs such as testes, uterus, heart, lungs or lead toxicity)[15]
- Late pregnancy
- High doses of ivermectin

High hematocrit/packed cell volume greater than 50%
- Dehydration
  - Gastric stasis
  - Trichoezoar (hair ball)
  - Malocclusion
- Shock (associated with splenic contraction).

Reduced total RBCs with increased nucleated RBCs
- Acute infection

Regenerative anemia
- Acute blood loss
- Chronic blood loss
  - Uterine adenocarcinoma
  - Endometrial hyperplasia
  - Gastric hemorrhage
  - Urolithiasis

Nonregenerative anemia signs
- Acute blood loss (initial stages)
- Lymphoma or chronic renal disease
- Chronic diseases
  - Pasteurellosis (snuffles)
  - Tracheobronchitis
  - Pododermatitis
  - Mastitis
  - Endometritis
  - Osteomyelitis
- Dental disease

Thrombocytes

Thrombocytopenia
- Acute infection
- Hemorrhage
- Inadequate mixing of a sample with an anticoagulant, resulting in microclots
- Disseminated intravascular coagulation (DIC)

Leukocytes

Leukopenia
- Chronic stress
- Acute infection
- Chronic infection

Neutrophilia
- Acute infection (with associated lymphopenia)

- o Pyogenic bacteria
- o Tissue inflammation/necrosis
- Prolonged stress
- Hyperadrenocorticism

Neutropenia
- Overwhelming acute or chronic bacterial infections
- Viral infections
- Hypersplenism
- Endotoxic, septic, or anaphylactic shock
- Estrogen producing tumors (eg, Sertoli cell tumor)
- Toxemia (uremia)
- Neoplasia

Lymphopenia
- Acute infection
- Stress
- Chronic exogenous steroid administration

Lymphophilia
- Lymphoma
- Viral infection

Eosinophilia
- Chronic parasitism
- Chronic skin disease or atopy (with associated basophilia)

Eosinopenia
- Chronic stress

Monocytosis
- Chronic infection
- Inflammation

REFERENCES

1. American Veterinary Medical Association. U.S. pet ownership & demographic sourcebook. Schaumberg (IL): AVMA; 2012.
2. Carpenter JW, Mashima TY, Gentz EJ, et al. Caring for rabbits: an overview and formulary. Vet Med 1995;90(4):340–64.
3. Hawk CT, Leary S. Formulary for laboratory animals. 3rd edition. Ames (IA): Wiley-Blackwell; 2005.
4. Dyer SM, Cervasio EL. An overview of restraint and blood collection techniques in exotic pet practice. Vet Clin North Am Exot Anim Pract 2008;11(3):423–43.
5. Murray MJ. Rabbit and ferret sampling and artifact considerations. In: Fudge AM, editor. Laboratory medicine avian and exotic pets. Philadelphia: Saunders; 2000. p. 265–8.
6. Mitruka BJ, Rawnsley HM. Clinical biochemical and hematological reference values in normal experimental animals. New York: Masson Publishing; 1977.

7. Ameri M, Schnaars HA, Sibley JR, et al. Stability of hematologic analytes in monkey, rabbit, rat, and mouse blood stored at 4°C in EDTA using the ADVIA 120 hematology analyzer. Vet Clin Pathol 2011;40(2):188–94.
8. Jain NC. Normal values in blood of laboratory, furbearing and miscellaneous zoo, domestic and wild animals. In: Jain NC, editor. Schalm's veterinary hematology. Philadelphia: Lea & Febiger; 1986. p. 274–343.
9. Hawkey CM, Dennett TB. Color atlas of comparative veterinary hematology. Ames (IA): Iowa State University Press; 1989.
10. Schermer S. The blood morphology of laboratory animals. Philadelphia: Davis Company; 1967.
11. Zimmerman KL, Moore DM, Smith ST. Hematology of laboratory rabbits. In: Weiss DJ, Wardrop KJ, editors. Schalm's, Veterinary Hematology. Philadelphia: Lippincott Williams and Wilkins; 2010. p. 862.
12. Balin A, Koren G, Hasu M, et al. Evaluation of a new method for the prevention of neonatal anemia. Pediatr Res 1989;25:274.
13. Bartolotti A, Castelli D, Bonati M. Hematology and serum chemistry of adult, pregnant, and newborn New Zealand rabbits (Oryctolagus cuniculus). Lab Anim Sci 1989;39:437.
14. Kozma C, Macklin LM, Cummins R, et al. Anatomy, physiology, and biochemistry of the rabbit. In: Weisbroth SH, Flatt RE, Kraus AL, editors. The biology of the laboratory rabbit. Orlando (FL): Academic Press; 1974. p. 64.
15. McLaughlin RM, Fish RE. Clinical biochemistry and hematology. In: Manning PJ, Ringler DH, Newcomer CE, editors. The biology of the laboratory rabbit. 2nd edition. San Diego (CA): Academic Press; 1994. p. 119–24.
16. Washington IM, Van Hoosier GM. Clinical biochemistry and hematology. In: Suckow MA, Stevens KA, Wilson RP, editors. The laboratory rabbit, guinea pig, hamster, and other rodents. Academic Press; 2012. p. 97–100.
17. Benson KG, Paul-Murphy J. Clinical pathology of the domestic rabbit. Vet Clin North Am Exot Anim Pract 1999;2(3). 542.
18. Reagan WJ, Irizarry Rovira AR, DeNicola DB, et al. Normal white cell morphology. In: Reagan WJ, Rovira ARI, DeNicola DB, editors. Veterinary hematology: atlas of common domestic and non-domestic species. Ames (IA): Blackwell; 2008. p. 29–35.
19. Etim NN, Williams ME, Akpabio U, et al. Haematological parameters and factors affecting their values. Agricultural Science 2014;2(1):40.
20. Marshall KL. Rabbit hematology. Vet Clin North Am Exot Anim Pract 2008;11: 551–67.
21. Nakyinsige K, Sazili AQ, Aghwan ZA, et al. Changes in blood constituents of rabbits subjected to transportation under hot, humid tropical conditions. Asian-Australas J Anim Sci 2013;26(6):874–8.
22. Costa-Freitas FL, Yamamoto BL, Freitas WL, et al. Systemic inflammatory response indicators in rabbits experimentally infected with sporulate oocysts of Eimeria sliedai. Rev Bras Parasitol Vet 2011;20(2):121–6.
23. Jacobson HA, Kirkpatrick RL, Burkhart HE, et al. Hematologic comparisons of shot and live trapped cottontail rabbits. J Wildl Dis 1978;14:82–8.
24. Kramp WJ. Herpesvirus sylvilagus infects both B and T lymphocytes in vivo. J Virol 1985;56(1):60–5.
25. Lepitzki DA, Woolf A. Hematology and serum chemistry of cottontail rabbits of southern Illinois. J Wildl Dis 1978;27(4):82–8.

Hematologic Assessment in Pet Rats, Mice, Hamsters, and Gerbils

Blood Sample Collection and Blood Cell Identification

Nicole M. Lindstrom, MS, DVM[a], David M. Moore, MS, DVM, DACLAM[a],*,
Kurt Zimmerman, DVM, PhD, DACVP[b], Stephen A. Smith, DVM, PhD[b]

KEYWORDS

- Hamster • Mouse • Rat • Gerbil • Blood collection • Hematology • Hemogram

KEY POINTS

- Hamsters, gerbils, rats, and mice are presented to veterinary clinics and hospitals for prophylactic care and treatment of clinical signs of disease.
- Normal reference hematologic parameters are valuable for comparison with the results of clinical and diagnostic testing, and for development of treatment plans for small rodent patients.
- It is important to recognize that several variables affect hemogram results, including methods of sample collection, preparation of samples, equipment, reagents, methods of analysis, age, gender, circadian rhythm, breed, and environment of the animals being sampled.

Medical treatment of pocket pets has become an increasing component of veterinary clinical practice. According to the 2013 to 2014 American Pet Products Association National Pet Owners Survey, 68% of US households own a pet, which is approximately 82.5 million homes. Roughly 6.9 million of those homes (8.3% of the total) owned noncat/nondog small animal species.[1] About 1.3 million households have small rodent species (rat, mouse, hamster, gerbil) as pets.[2]

Normal reference hematologic parameters are valuable for comparison with the results of clinical and diagnostic testing, and for development of treatment plans for

[a] Virginia Tech, 300 Turner Street Northwest, Suite 4120 (0497), Blacksburg, VA 24061, USA;
[b] Department of Biomedical Sciences and Pathobiology (0442), Virginia-Maryland Regional College of Veterinary Medicine, 245 Duck Pond Drive, Blacksburg, VA 24061, USA
* Corresponding author.
E-mail address: moored@vt.edu

Vet Clin Exot Anim 18 (2015) 21–32
http://dx.doi.org/10.1016/j.cvex.2014.09.004
1094-9194/15/$ – see front matter © 2015 Elsevier Inc. All rights reserved.

small rodent patients. It is important to recognize that several variables affect hemogram results, including methods of sample collection, preparation of samples, equipment, reagents, methods of analysis, age, gender, circadian rhythm, breed, and environment of the animals being sampled.[3,4] As a resource for veterinarians and their technicians, this article describes the methods for collection of blood, identification of blood cells, and interpretation of the hemogram in mice, rats, gerbils and hamsters.

BIOSAFETY AND OCCUPATIONAL HEALTH CONSIDERATIONS FOR CLINIC STAFF

Rodents from pet stores, from the wild, and pet rodents that may be exposed to wild rodents in the home, can carry several zoonotic diseases that can be easily transmitted to humans. A variety of publications are available that explain in detail the signs and symptoms of these diseases in both rodents and humans.[5–8] Zoonotic agents of concern are listed in **Table 1**, along with the modes of transmission, clinical signs in animals, and symptoms in humans.

Of equal importance for occupational safety in the clinic when handling small pet rodents is the recognition that these rodents produce allergens that can cause acute allergic reactions in handlers (dermatologic, such as wheal-and-flare reaction; eye and nasal passage irritation); in hypersensitized individuals there is a risk of anaphylactic shock. Allergens are secreted in the urine and saliva of rats, mice, and gerbils. It should be recognized that fur and dander may be contaminated with the allergens from grooming (saliva) or contact with urine in the cage environment.

Exposure risks for clinic staff can be mitigated by appropriate handling and restraint of the animals, wearing basic personal protective equipment (gloves, mask, long-sleeved coat or gown, eye protection), practicing good personal hygiene, sanitization of examination room surfaces the rodents came into contact with, and effective rodent pest control in the clinic.[5]

METHODOLOGY FOR BLOOD COLLECTION
Restraint

Proper restraint is an absolute necessity for venipuncture of small mammals. Most hamsters, gerbils, mice, and rats can undergo manual restraint alone for venipuncture. However, it is important to remember that the handling and restraint, transport to the veterinary hospital, and the hospital environment itself are stressful to these prey species. It is vital to approach these animals calmly and confidently and to minimize visual, olfactory, and auditory stimuli.[3,9,10] Anesthesia may be needed for adequate restraint to obtain samples from small mammals. However, anesthesia itself has been shown to produce changes in hematology parameters including decreased hematocrit, hemoglobin level, and red blood cell (RBC) count.[3] Handling and restraint, sedation, and anesthetic protocols for mice, rats, hamsters, and gerbils have been described in a variety of articles and books.[11–15]

Manual restraint
Mice Pet mice that are accustomed to being held can be lifted with both hands. To move single animals for short periods of time (2–3 seconds) from cage to examination table, grasp the animal gently at the base of the tail and lift. Do not lift mice by the tip of their tail, because that results in degloving injuries to the tail tip. The other hand can be placed under the mouse for additional support. Alternatively, mice can be picked up by the base of the tail or scruff of the neck using rubber-tipped forceps. Mice can also be coaxed, head first, into an appropriately sized disposable plastic syringe cover or large centrifuge tube, leaving the tail exposed for blood collection.

Table 1
Zoonotic disease agents in small rodents

Pathogen	Transmission	Animal Disease	Human Disease
Streptobacillus moniliformis, *Spirillum minor* (rat bite fever, Haverhill fever)	Animal bites, ingestion of contaminated food products	Usually a subclinical infection, but purulent lesions have been reported in some animals	Polyarthritis, myalgias, regional lymphadenopathy, fever
Salmonellosis (most rodents)	Fecal-oral, ingestion of contaminated products	Malaise, dehydration, bloody diarrhea	Dehydration, vomiting, abdominal pain, nausea
Leptospirosis (most rodents)	Direct contact with contaminated urine	Infertility, fever, anorexia, anemia	Headache, myalgia, conjunctivitis, nausea
Lymphocytic choriomeningitis	Exposure to saliva or urine from infected animals or to infected cell lines in the laboratory. Fomites may play a role	Viremia, viuria, and chronic wasting disease	Subclinical infection, mild flulike symptoms. Viral meningitis and encephalitis (rare)
Hantavirus (most rodents)	Exposure to aerosols, urine, and fecal material from infected animals. Fomites may play a role	Subclinical	Fever, myalgia, petechiation, abdominal pain, headache
Dermatophytosis (*Trichophyton mentagrophytes*)	Direct contact	Circular raised erythematous lesion with hyperkeratosis and hair loss	Circular raised erythematous lesions with hyperkeratosis and hair loss
Ornythonysisus bacoti (tropical rat mite)	Direct contact with cage materials	Asymptomatic to moderate pruritus	Severe pruritus
Sarcoptes scabei (guinea pigs and hamsters)	Direct contact with infected animal	Intense pruritus	Intense pruritus

Restraint for performing an examination, treatments, or procedures has been described in detail elsewhere.[16] Briefly, restraint can be performed by hand or using a commercially available restraint device. To restrain a mouse by hand, grasp the tail at its base with the nondominant hand and lift the mouse onto the cage lid or similar rough surface. If gentle traction is kept on the tail base, the animal moves forward and grasps onto the cage lid or other surface with its forepaws. The handler can tuck the base of the tail between the third and fourth finger, and then firmly grasp the mouse by the scruff with the same hand that is holding the tail. Gathering sufficient skin in the scruff-hold prevents the mouse from twisting or turning such that it can bite the handler. Recognize that drawing up loose skin in the scruff-hold can leave little room for respiratory movements of the ribs, which can result in asphyxiation of the mouse. The scruff-hold, therefore, should be used for only brief periods of time, and the handler should observe the pinna, nose, and paws for signs of cyanosis.

Rats Large pet rats should be restrained using an over- or under-the-shoulders grip with the thumb and fingers of one hand (thoracic encirclement), or using a commercially available restraint device or towel.[16] The over-the-shoulder grip can be performed by grasping the rat by the base of the tail and pulling gently backward with the dominant hand. Then place the nondominant hand over the back of the rat and grasp the rat around the thorax with the head of the rat between the index and middle fingers. It is important to not overcompress the rat's thorax and prevent respiratory movements of the ribs, resulting in anoxia. The body of the rat can then be stabilized by the handler's other hand, arm, or body. The under-the-shoulders grip is performed similarly, except the rat is grasped around the thorax, immediately under the shoulder blades. The forearms of the rat are gently pushed cranially with the thumb and index finger, and they cross under the chin, preventing the animal from biting the handler. Commercially available plastic restraint devices are very useful when performing blood draws on rats. Rats may be restrained in other ways, such as by wrapping in a small towel, or by simply cupping a hand over the animal.[16]

Gerbils Gerbils are usually docile animals and can simply be picked up and carefully restrained by the skin over the scruff of the neck. The gerbil can also be enclosed within one hand and held firmly in an upright position. Gerbils should not be picked up by the tip of the tail because of the risk of degloving injury.[12,17,18]

Hamsters Hamsters can be docile when handled frequently but care must be taken to avoid being bitten. To avoid startling a sleeping hamster before restraint, talk to the animal and gently touch its body one or two times to ensure that it is awake and aware of the handler's presence. Manual restraint of hamsters can be performed by gathering the loose skin over the scruff of the neck in one hand. Loose skin may be an understatement—there is generally enough skin that you could put in another two hamsters. In contrast to the scruff-hold in rats, mice, and gerbils, great care should be taken to gather enough of the hamster's loose skin into the scruff-hold such that the corners of the mouth are drawn back into a smile (a "smiling" hamster is one that cannot bite the handler). A hamster can also be placed in an appropriately sized plastic restraint tube for blood collection. These tubes should have air holes at the nose end, and be cleaned frequently to reduce the risk of cross-infection or stress from pheromones.[12,17,19]

Chemical restraint
Drugs that can be used for sedation, tranquilization, and anesthesia of mice, rats, hamsters, and gerbils have been described in published literature, and many online

formularies for injectable anesthesia are available.[15,20] Inhalant anesthesia (isoflurane) is frequently used for rapid induction and anesthesia of small pet rodents.

Blood Collection Sites in Rats, Mice, Gerbils, and Hamsters: Location, Preparation, and Venipuncture Techniques

Several references are available that describe blood collection techniques in small pet rodents.[11–13] Recommended venipuncture sites for small pet rodents, used in clinical practice, are summarized in **Table 2**. A representative cross-section of a rodent's tail is provided in **Fig. 1**. Blood can be collected from the lateral tail veins and ventral caudal artery of mice, rats, and gerbils.

Collection from tail veins

The lateral tail veins run the length of the tail, and are more readily visualized in nonpigmented animals.[21] Vasodilation can be induced by placing the animal in an isolator at 104°F for a few minutes, or applying a warm water compress. "Milking" the vein, applying slight compression and stroking from base to tip, in an attempt to dilate the vessels, should not be done because this results in leukocytosis of the sample. After swabbing the venipuncture site with an appropriate disinfectant, a sterile hypodermic needle or a sterile lancet is used to prick the vein, and blood is collected in a microhematocrit tube or a microcentrifuge containing an appropriate volume of anticoagulant. Gentle pressure should be applied over the venipuncture site to stop the bleeding.

Collection from ventral caudal artery

This artery runs the length of the tail, but is not readily visualized. After the collection site has been disinfected, a 23- to 25-gauge needle (the smaller size for smaller species) is inserted in the ventral midline, about one-third the length of the tail from the body. The needle is inserted at a 30-degree angle, in a cranial direction, until it contacts the bone of the ventral surface of the caudal vertebra. The needle is then slightly withdrawn until blood begins to flow through the needle, and then is maintained in that position. Blood

Table 2 Recommended venipuncture sites in small pet rodent	
Species	**Vessel**
Mouse	Lateral saphenous vein Femoral vein Medial saphenous vein Jugular vein Lateral tail vein Ventral tail artery Facial vein (superficial temporal)
Rat	Saphenous vein Femoral vein Jugular vein Dorsal and lateral tail veins Ventral tail artery Cranial vena cava
Gerbil	Saphenous vein Metatarsal vein Lateral tail vein
Hamster	Lateral saphenous vein Cephalic vein Cranial vena cava

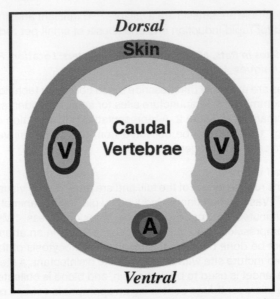

Fig. 1. Cross-section of rodent tail, showing vessels used for blood collection.

can be collected in a microhematocrit tube as it flows from the needle hub. In rats, a 1- or 3-mL syringe, with its plunger removed, can be affixed to the needle before arterial puncture is attempted, and blood is allowed to flow into the barrel of the syringe. After blood collection, gentle pressure should be applied to the arterial puncture site for several minutes to prevent continued blood flow.

Collection from hindlimb vessels
Blood can be collected from the lateral saphenous veins[22] and dorsal metatarsal veins of mice, rats, hamsters, and gerbils. The anatomic locations and procedures for blood collection from those vessels are provided in the article on guinea pig hematology elsewhere in this issue.

Blood can be collected from the facial vein after pricking it with a sterile lancet.[23] This technique has been used successfully in rats, mice, hamsters, and gerbils used in research. However, this method requires practice to accomplish successfully, and practice animals are generally not readily available in most veterinary practices. Thus the procedure has been referenced, but is not described herein.

Blood Volume Collected
Blood collection from small mammals is challenging because of limited blood volume available for sampling, and because the restraint or sedation necessary to obtain a sample may alter the results of some assays.[3,4,11,12,18] The maximum volume of blood that can be safely withdrawn in a single sample is approximately 7.5% to 10% of the circulating blood volume.[11] **Table 3** provides information to assist in determining the maximum safe blood sample volume in small pet rodents based on the animal's body weight. It is important to adhere to these recommended limits to prevent hypovolemic shock and anemia. The extracted volume is replaced within 24 hours in most healthy animals, although a return to normal levels of all blood constituents may take up to 2 weeks.[11] The volume and frequency of blood collection must also take into account the health status of the patient.

Table 3 Determining maximum safe blood sample volumes in small rodents based on body weight		
Body Weight (g)	Circulating Blood Volume (mL)	Draw No More than 7.5%–10% of Circulating Blood Volume (mL)
20	1.10–1.40	0.082–0.14
25	1.37–1.75	0.10–0.18
30	1.65–2.10	0.12–0.21
35	1.93–2.45	0.14–0.25
40	2.20–2.80	0.16–0.28
125	6.88–8.75	0.52–0.88
150	8.25–10.50	0.62–1.0
200	11.00–14.00	0.82–1.4
250	13.75–17.50	1.0–1.8
300	16.50–21.00	1.2–2.1
350	19.25–24.50	1.4–2.5

Data from National Institutes of Health. NIH guidelines for survival bleeding of rats and mice. 2012.

MORPHOLOGY AND NUMBERS OF PERIPHERAL BLOOD CELLS

Referenced ranges of hematologic parameters in normal rats, mice, hamsters, and gerbils are provided in **Table 4**. Values listed for hamsters are for the Syrian (golden) hamster. Hematologic values for European and Djungarian hamsters have been described in the literature.[27–29] Reference values should be used as a tool for diagnosis and treatment, along with clinical signs and physical examination parameters, but not as the sole guide to determine if values are normal or abnormal.[3,4,11,12]

Erythrocytes

The approximate diameters of erythrocytes in small rodents are as follows: mouse, 5 to 7 μm; rat, 5.7 to 7 μm; and hamster, 5 to 7 μm.[3] Moderate anisocytosis is seen in mouse, rat, and hamster RBCs, with the diameter of some cells only one-third that of the standard RBC size. In rats and mice, Howell-Jolly bodies and nucleated RBCs are sometimes observed. RBCs of young rats and mice are morphologically variable, and young animals have more circulating reticulocytes than do older animals (10%–20% vs 2%–5%).[3] Neonatal gerbils have erythrocyte counts that are approximately one-half adult values, but increase to adult values by about 8 weeks of age.[9] Gerbils up to 20 weeks old have a large number of circulating reticulocytes and erythrocytes with basophilic stippling and polychromasia. These cells are also abundant in older gerbils and are probably associated with the short erythrocyte lifespan.[9] The lifespan of erythrocytes in small rodents is as follows: mouse, 41 to 52 days; rat, 56 to 69 days; hamster, 50 to 78 days; and gerbil, 10 days.[3] Hibernation (more correctly, pseudohibernation) in hamsters prolongs the life span of their erythrocytes. The end of hibernation in the hamster is associated with an increase in reticulocyte numbers.[3] Comparative values of erythrocyte numbers are provided in **Table 4**.

Thrombocytes (Platelets)

The mouse thrombocyte is round to oval to elongated in shape, and approximately 1 to 4 μm in diameter. Rat and mouse platelets have similar morphology. Round

Table 4
Referenced ranges of hematologic parameters in normal rats, mice, hamsters, and gerbils

	Rat		Mouse		Hamster		Gerbil	
	Male	Female	Male	Female	Male	Female	Male	Female
RBC ($\times 10^6$/μL)	8.15–9.75	6.76–9.2	6.9–11.7	6.86–11.3	4.7–10.3	3.96–9.96	7.1–8.6	8.0–9.4
PCV (%)	44.4–50.4	37.6–50.6	33.1–49.9	39.7–44.5	47.9–57.1	39.2–58.8	42–49	43–50
Hgb (g/dL)	13.4–15.8	11.5–16.1	11.1–11.5	10.7–11.1	14.4–19.2	13.1–18.9	12.1–13.8	13.1–16.9
MCV (fL)	49.8–57.8	50.9–65.5	47.5–50.5	47–52	64.8–77.6	64–76	46.6–60	46.64–60.04
MCH (pg)	14.3–18.3	15.6–19	11.7–12.7	11.1–12.7	19.9–24.9	20.2–25.8	16.1–19.4	16.3–19.4
MCHC (%)	26.2–35.4	26.5–36.1	23.2–31.2	22.3–29.5	27.5–36.5	27.8–37.4	30.6–33.3	30.6–33.3
Platelets ($\times 10^3$/μL)	150–450	160–460	157–412	170–410	367–573	300–490	432–710	540–632
WBC ($\times 10^3$/μL)	8.0–11.8	6.6–12.6	12.5–15.9	12.1–13.7	5.02–10.2	6.48–10.6	4.3–12.3	5.6–12.8
Neutrophils (%)	6.2–42.6	4.4–49.2	13.2–21.6	15.7–18.5	17.1–27.1	22.8–35.2	9.3–23.6	10.7–25.8
Lymphocytes (%)	57.6–83.2	50.2–84.5	62.4–82.8	65.9–77.9	54.7–92.3	50.9–84.9	68–76.8	58.9–78.1
Eosinophils (%)	0.1–0.63	0–1.96	1.37–2.81	2.05–2.77	0.26–1.54	0.22–1.18	0–1.6	0–2.3
Basophils (%)	0–0.6	0–0.4	0.22–0.82	0.13–0.85	0–5	0–2.1	0–1.6	0–0.8
Monocytes (%)	0–0.65	0–1.81	2.22–2.47	0.98–1.11	0.9–4.1	0.4–4.4	0–6.5	1.7–6.2

Abbreviations: Hgb, hemoglobin; MCH, mean corpuscular hemoglobin; MCHC, mean corpuscular hemoglobin concentration; MCV, mean corpuscular volume; PCV, packed cell volume.
Data from Refs.[9,24–26]

platelets the size of RBCs and platelet clumps may be frequently observed.[3] The margins of platelets appear indistinct in Wright-Giemsa–stained blood smears.[3] The cytoplasm of mouse and rat thrombocytes has a faint pink to gray color, and toward the center of the cell, blue angular granules may be observed, and occasionally red granules may be present.[3] In hamsters, platelets appear to be amorphous veils of a gray-blue ground substance with violet-stained granules.[9,30] Comparative values of thrombocyte numbers are provided in **Table 4**.

Leukocytes (White Blood Cells)

Leukocyte concentrations in these small pet rodents demonstrate diurnal variation,[3] and thus laboratory results are affected by the time of day when the sample is collected.

Acute stress in rats results in elevated serum corticosterone but with a normal neutrophil/lymphocyte ratio, whereas chronic stress (distress) yields the opposite— normal serum corticosterone concentrations with an elevated neutrophil/lymphocyte ratio.[31] Although neutrophilia and lymphopenia were seen in chronically stressed rats, the values for each were with normal referenced ranges.[31] A similar picture is seen in aging mice and rats, when the proportion of lymphocytes decreases and the proportion of neutrophils increases.[3]

The ranges of total WBC numbers and the white blood cell (WBC) types observed in a standard differential count are provided in **Table 4**. Typical WBCs for each of the small pet rodents are provided in the following figures: mouse WBCs (**Fig. 2**), rat WBCs (**Fig. 3**), hamster WBCs (**Fig. 4**), and gerbil WBCs (**Fig. 5**).

Neutrophils

The nucleus of the neutrophil in rodents has several indentations, giving it a hyperseg-mented appearance. Band forms may be seen in normal animals, but this is usually seen in association with inflammation.[3] Ring forms may be seen, but are usually associated with accelerated ganulopoiesls.[3] The cytoplasm of neutrophils is pale with faint pink granules. In hamsters, neutrophils (heterophils) resemble eosinophils, with a lobular nucleus and dense pink cytoplasmic granules. Comparative values of neutrophils observed in differential counts in normal mice, rats, hamsters, and gerbils are provided in **Table 4**.

Lymphocytes

In mice, rats, hamsters, and gerbils, lymphocytes comprise approximately 75% of the leukocytes in the peripheral blood. Lymphocytes in rats and mice may be small or large with variable amounts of cytoplasm, varying from deep to pale blue, and sometimes containing large, dark-staining, azurophilic granules. In hamsters, lymphocytes are small round cells with a dark blue nucleus that fills most of the cell and is

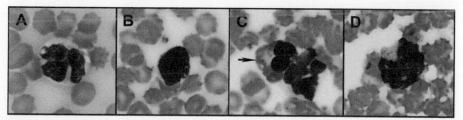

Fig. 2. Representative mouse blood cells. (*A*) Neutrophil and RBCs. (*B*) Lymphocyte and RBCs. (*C*) Eosinophil and RBCs. (*D*) Monocyte and RBCs. The *arrow* is pointing out the eosin-ophil. (Wright-Giemsa stain; 1000x).

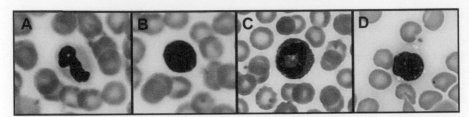

Fig. 3. Representative rat blood cells. (*A*) Neutrophil and RBCs. (*B*) Lymphocyte and RBCs. (*C*) Eosinophil and RBCs. (*D*) Monocyte, platelet, and RBCs. (Wright-Giemsa stain; 1000x).

surrounded by a rim of lighter blue cytoplasm. Comparative values of lymphocytes observed in differential counts in normal mice, rats, hamsters, and gerbils are provided in **Table 4**.

Eosinophils
In mice, eosinophils have a band-shaped and occasionally ring-shaped nucleus that is partially obscured by the presence of ruddy orange to red granules. The granules are large, round, and fairly uniform in size, but have indistinct borders.[3] In rats, eosinophils have nuclei that are usually less segmented than neutrophils and contain small, round, reddish granules that fill the cytoplasm. In hamsters, the nucleus is annual-shaped, sometimes twisted, that fills the periphery of the call as a wide band. The nucleus is surrounded by a narrow zone of cytoplasm, which is tightly packed with rod-shaped azurophilic granules.[3] Comparative values of eosinophils observed in differential counts in normal mice, rats, hamsters, and gerbils are provided in **Table 4**.

Basophils
In rats, mice, and hamsters, basophils are rarely observed on peripheral blood smears. They lack tertiary granules but have larger and less numerous mature granules. Basophil nuclei are lobulated, and the cytoplasm contains large, round purple granules that may be few in number or so numerous that they obscure the nucleus. Comparative values of basophils observed in differential counts in normal mice, rats, hamsters, and gerbils are provided in **Table 4**.

Monocytes
Monocytes are the largest-sized WBC in these small rodents. Monocyte morphology is similar to that seen in other species with pleomorphic nuclei that may be round, indented, or lobular, an extensive cytoplasm that stains pale gray blue, and often

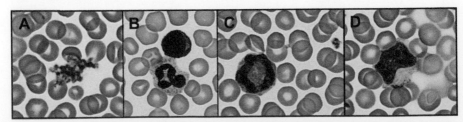

Fig. 4. Representative hamster blood cells. (*A*) Clumped platelets and RBCs. (*B*) Neutrophil, lymphocyte, and RBCs. (*C*) Eosinophil, platelet, and RBCs. (*D*) Monocyte and RBCs. (Wright-Giemsa stain; 1000x).

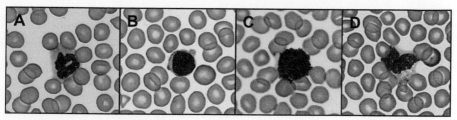

Fig. 5. Representative gerbil blood cells. (*A*) Neutrophil and RBCs. (*B*) Lymphocyte and RBCs. (*C*) Basophil and RBCs. (*D*) Monocyte and RBCs. (Wright-Giemsa stain; 1000x).

contains vacuoles.[3] Comparative values of monocytes observed in differential counts in normal mice, rats, hamsters, and gerbils are provided in **Table 4**.

REFERENCES

1. American Pet Products Association. 2013–2014 National Pet Owners Survey. Greenwich (CT): American Pet Products Manufacturers Association; 2014.
2. American Veterinary Medical Association. 2012 U.S. pet ownership & demographic sourcebook. Schaumberg (IL): AVMA; 2012.
3. Provencher Bollinger A, Everds NE, Zimmerman KL. Hematology of laboratory animals. In: Weiss DJ, Wardrop KJ, editors. Schalm's veterinary hematology. Philadelphia: Lippincott Williams and Wilkins; 2010. p. 852–62.
4. Washington IM, Van Hoosier G. Clinical biochemistry and hematology. In: Suckow MA, Stevens KA, Wilson RP, editors. The laboratory rabbit, guinea pig, hamster, and other rodents. 1st edition. London: Academic Press; 2012. p. 57–116.
5. Hill WA, Brown JP. Zoonoses of rabbits and rodents. Vet Clin North Am Exot Anim Pract 2011;14(3):519–31, vii.
6. Chomel BB. Zoonoses of house pets other than dogs, cats and birds. Pediatr Infect Dis J 1992;11:479–87.
7. American Biological Safety Association. Zoonotic diseases fact sheet. Mundelein (IL): ABSA; 2012.
8. Committee on Occupational Health and Safety in Research Animals Facilities, Institute of Laboratory Animal Resources, Commission of Life Sciences, National Research Council. Occupational health and safety in the care and use of research animals. Washington, DC: National Academic Press; 1997.
9. Zimmerman KL, Moore DM, Smith SA. Hematology of the Mongolian gerbil. In: Weiss DJ, Wardrop KJ, editors. Schalm's veterinary hematology. Philadelphia: Lippincott Williams and Wilkins; 2010. p. 899–903.
10. Smith SA, Zimmerman KL, Moore DM. Hematology of the Syrian (golden) hamster. In: Weiss DJ, Wardrop KJ, editors. Schalm's veterinary hematology. Philadelphia: Lippincott Williams and Wilkins; 2010. p. 904–9.
11. Ott Joslin J. Blood collection techniques in small mammals. J Exotic Pet Medicine 2009;18:117–39.
12. Hrapkiewicz K, Colby L, Denison P. Clinical laboratory animal medicine: an introduction. 4th edition. Ames (IA): Wiley Blackwell; 2013.
13. Dyer SM, Cervasio EL. An overview of restraint and blood collection techniques in exotic pet practice. Vet Clin North Am Exot Anim Pract 2008;11(3):423–43.
14. Fowler ME. Restraint and handling of wild and domestic animals. 3rd edition. Ames (IA): Wiley-Blackwell; 2008.

15. Longley LA. Anesthesia of exotic pets. Philadelphia: Saunders Elsevier; 2008.
16. Machholz E, Mulder G, Ruiz C, et al. Manual restraint and common compound administration routes in mice and rats. J Vis Exp 2012;(67):e2771. http://dx.doi.org/10.3791/2771.
17. Harkness JE, Wagner JE. The biology and medicine of rabbits and rodents. 4th edition. Baltimore (MD): Williams and Wilkins; 1995.
18. Batchelder M, Keller LS, Sauer MB, et al. Gerbils. In: Suckow MA, Stevens KA, Wilson RP, editors. The laboratory rabbit, guinea pig, hamster, and other rodents. 1st edition. London: Academic Press; 2012. p. 1131–55.
19. Fenyk-Melody J. The European hamster. In: Suckow MA, Stevens KA, Wilson RP, editors. The laboratory rabbit, guinea pig, hamster, and other rodents. 1st edition. London: Academic Press; 2012. p. 923–33.
20. Hawk CT, Leary S. Formulary for laboratory animals. 3rd edition. Ames (IA): Wiley-Blackwell; 2005.
21. Brown C. Blood collection from the tail of a rat. Lab Anim (NY) 2006;35(8):24–5.
22. Hem A, Smith AJ, Solberg P. Saphenous vein puncture for blood sampling of the mouse, rat, hamster, gerbil, guinea pig, ferret and mink. Lab Anim 1998;32(4):364–8.
23. Golde WT, Gollobin P, Rodriguez LL. A rapid, simple, and humane method for submandibular bleeding of mice using a lancet. Lab Anim (NY) 2005;34:39–43.
24. Mitruka BJ, Rawnsley HM. Clinical biochemical and hematological reference values in normal experimental animals. New York: Masson Publishing; 1977. p. 82–3.
25. Mays A Jr. Baseline hematological and blood biochemical parameters of the Mongolian gerbil (Meriones unguiculatus). Lab Anim Care 1969;19:838–42.
26. Ruhren R. Normal values for hemoglobin concentration and cellular elements in the blood of Mongolian gerbils. Lab Anim Care 1965;15:313–20.
27. Mitchell MA, Tully TN. Manual of exotic pet practice. St Louis (MO): Saunders Elsevier; 2009. p. 414.
28. Moore DM. Hematology of the Syrian (golden) hamster (Mesocricetus auratus). In: Feldman BF, Zinkl JG, Jain NC, editors. Schalm's veterinary hematology. 5th edition. Philadelphia: Lippincott Williams & Wilkins; 2000. p. 1115–9.
29. Moore DM. Hematology of the Mongolian gerbil (Meriones unguiculatus). In: Feldman BF, Zinkl JG, Jain NC, editors. Schalm's veterinary hematology. 5th edition. Philadelphia: Lippincott Williams & Wilkins; 2000. p. 1111–4.
30. Schermer S. The blood morphology of laboratory animals. 3rd edition. Philadelphia: FA Davis; 1967.
31. Swan MP, Hickman DL. Evaluation of the neutrophil-lymphocyte ratio as a measure of distress in rats. Lab Anim (NY) 2014;43(8):276–82.

Hematological Assessment in Pet Guinea Pigs (*Cavia porcellus*)

Blood Sample Collection and Blood Cell Identification

Kurt Zimmerman, DVM, PhD, DACVP[a],*, David M. Moore, MS, DVM, DACLAM[b],
Stephen A. Smith, DVM, MS, PhD[a]

KEYWORDS

- Guinea pig • Guinea pig blood collection • Guinea pig hematology
- Guinea pig hemogram • Guinea pig WBC morphology • Guinea pig differential count

KEY POINTS

- Pet guinea pigs are presented to veterinary clinics for routine care and treatment of clinical diseases.
- In addition to obtaining clinical history and physical exam findings, diagnostic testing may be required, including hematological assessments.
- Guinea pigs are subject to dental problems (malocclusion), nutritional problems (vitamin C deficiency), bacterial infections (cervical lymphadenitis, pneumonia), reproductive/metabolic problems (dystocia, pregnancy toxemia), internal and external parasites, and musculoskeletal problems (fracture of the spine), some of which may require hematological assessment by veterinary clinicians.

Approximately 1.3 million guinea pigs are maintained as pets in about 0.84 million homes in the United States.[1] They have a long lifespan (5–7 years)[2,3] compared with other, smaller rodents, and are more likely to be presented for clinical care than other rodent species. Guinea pigs are subject to dental problems (malocclusion), nutritional problems (vitamin C deficiency), bacterial infections (cervical lymphadenitis, pneumonia), reproductive/metabolic problems (dystocia, pregnancy toxemia), internal and external parasites, and musculoskeletal problems (fracture of the spine),

---

[a] Department of Biomedical Sciences and Pathobiology (0442), Virginia-Maryland Regional College of Veterinary Medicine, Duck Pond Drive, Blacksburg, VA 24061, USA; [b] Department of Biomedical Sciences and Pathobiology, Virginia Tech, 300 Turner Street Northwest, Suite 4120 (0497), Blacksburg, VA 24061, USA
* Corresponding author.
E-mail address: kzimmerm@vt.edu

Vet Clin Exot Anim 18 (2015) 33–40
http://dx.doi.org/10.1016/j.cvex.2014.09.002
1094-9194/15/$ – see front matter © 2015 Elsevier Inc. All rights reserved.

some of which may require hematological assessment by veterinary clinicians. As a resource for veterinarians and their technicians, this article describes the methods for manual restraint, collection of blood, and identification of blood cells in guinea pigs.

METHODOLOGY FOR BLOOD COLLECTION
Restraint

Although guinea pigs may be naturally curious, they dislike change (eg, changes in diet, environment, handlers, unfamiliar noise), and may make an attempt to flee to avoid restraint. Some people refer to them as whistle pigs, because they make high-pitched vocalizations when excited or frightened; this sound should not be interpreted as pain when standard, nonpainful procedures, including manual restraint, are used. Some handlers abandon efforts to restrain a vocalizing animal for fear of causing harm, even though the restraint is needed for proper clinical diagnosis and treatment of the animal.

The handler should not attempt to restrain or pick up the animal by grasping the skin over the scruff of the neck; that is distressing to the animal, and should not be attempted. When picking up the guinea pig for examination or to move it from one area to another, the handler should place one hand over the dorsum, behind the shoulders, and grasp the animal gently but securely with the thumb and fingers around the rib cage, taking care not to restrict respiratory movements of the ribs. When lifting the animal, the other hand should be placed under the hindquarters for support. If the hindquarters are not supported, the animal may struggle and twist, causing injury to the spine, with resultant paresis or paralysis of the hind limbs.

Guinea pigs may become distressed if restrained in lateral or dorsal recumbency.[4] Guinea pigs may be wrapped securely in a towel, which seems to calm or comfort them. However, swaddling a guinea pig tends to make most vessels used for venipuncture inaccessible. Thus, additional care should be taken when wrapping the animal to allow access to the intended venipuncture site.

Compared with other pet rodent species and rabbits, the guinea pig is unlikely to bite the handler.

Drugs that can be used in sedation, tranquilization, and anesthesia of guinea pigs have been described in published literature.[5–7] However, professional judgment should be used to assess whether it is safe, based on the animal's clinical status, to anesthetize the animal.

Blood Collection Sites: Location and Preparation, and Venipuncture Techniques

Several veins are used as common venipuncture sites in guinea pigs, including the lateral saphenous and metatarsal veins of the hind limbs, and the cephalic veins of the forelegs.[8–10] Additional methods include the jugular vein, cranial vena cava, femoral vein, pricking a tiny vein in the pinna, or close clipping of a nail. **Table 1** provides a comparison of the advantages and disadvantages of the various blood collection sites in guinea pigs.

Given the small diameters of the commonly used veins, the phlebotomist should select an appropriately sized needle (eg, 22–30 gauge).

To induce vasodilation and facilitate blood collection, the animal can be placed in an incubator with an internal temperature of 40°C (104°F) for several minutes. As an alternative, an examination glove can be filled with water, tied off, microwaved until its temperature is warm but not scalding to the touch, and applied to the venipuncture site for about a minute.

Table 1
Comparison of blood collection sites in the guinea pig

Collection Site	Advantages	Disadvantages
Lateral saphenous vein	• Easily visualized • Easily accessible • Does not require sedation/anesthesia • Good for collecting small to moderate volumes of blood	• The vein is small and easily collapsed with rapid aspiration • Restraint may injure leg
Lateral metatarsal vein	• Easily visualized • Easily accessible • Does not require sedation/anesthesia • Good for collecting small volumes of blood	• The vein is small and easily collapsed with rapid aspiration • Restraint may injure leg • Free-flow sample is not sterile
Cephalic vein	• Good for collecting small volumes of blood	• Vein is mobile, requires stabilization • Vein may collapse during aspiration • Forelimb is short, making access difficult
Cranial vena cava	• Good for collecting moderate volumes of blood	• Cannot be visualized or palpated; rely on landmarks • Sedation/anesthesia required • Risk of internal bleeding
Jugular vein	• Good for collecting moderate volumes of blood	• Cannot be visualized or palpated; rely on landmarks • Sedation/anesthesia recommended • May become dyspneic when the neck is extended back during restraint
Ear veins	• Easily visualized • Easily accessible • Does not require sedation/anesthesia • Collecting small volumes of blood	• Could be irritating/painful • Free-flow sample is not sterile
Toenail clip	• Easily visualized • Easily accessible • Does not require sedation/anesthesia • Collecting small volumes of blood	• Could be irritating/painful • Free-flow sample is not sterile

Fig. 1 shows the location of the primary venipuncture sites on the hind limb. The fur over the selected site should be removed with electric clippers, and the site swabbed with an appropriate disinfectant solution.

The lateral saphenous vein runs dorsoventrally and then laterally over the tarsal joint. The foot should be grasped and traction applied to extend the leg. An assistant should apply digital pressure, gently squeezing the leg between the thumb and forefinger, proximal to the venipuncture site. Blood collection may be accomplished using a needle and syringe, or the vessel may be pricked/punctured using a sterile needle or

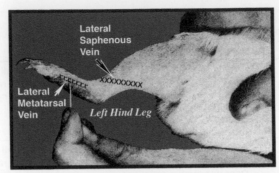

Fig. 1. Location of the lateral saphenous and lateral metatarsal veins in the guinea pig.

sterile lancet.[11] With the needle-and-syringe method, a needle of 23 to 25 gauge on a 1.0-mL syringe is inserted in the vein in a distal to proximal direction and, with slow aspiration to avoid collapse of the vessel, about 0.5 to 1.0 mL of blood can be collected.[4] For the free-flow method, pressure is applied (as described earlier) to dilate the vein, then a sterile needle of 20 to 23 gauge or a sterile lancet can be used to prick the vessel, with from 0.1 to 3 mL of blood collected in a microhematocrit tube, Pasteur pipette, or a snap-cap microcentrifuge tube that contains an appropriate volume of anticoagulant solution. Following either collection method, gentle pressure should be applied to the venipuncture site to stop the flow of blood and to prevent hematoma formation.

The lateral metatarsal vein is located on the lateral aspect of the foot. Preparation of the venipuncture site is the same as described earlier. Free-flow collection of blood from this vein and prevention of hematoma formation is also as described earlier. From 0.1 to 3 mL of blood may be collected by this method.[4,12] The dorsal metatarsal vein (not shown) may also be used for blood collection, using the techniques described earlier.

The procedure for cephalic venipuncture is similar to that in dogs and cats, but is more difficult because of the short length of the guinea pig forearm.

A small free-flow sample of blood may be collected by pricking/puncturing one of the small veins in the pinna, using appropriate presampling and postsampling procedures as described earlier.

Clipping a toenail to the quick yields some blood, but the procedure is painful and may lead to a secondary infection in the nail.

Volume Collected

In general, up to 50 µL of blood can collected in a microhematocrit tube from the saphenous vein, metatarsal vein, ear veins, or clipped toenail in adult guinea pigs.[13] Larger volumes of blood may be collected, within a range of 0.5 to 0.7 mL/100 g of body weight.[4,8,14] That range is based on the consensus that 7% to 10% of blood volume can safely be collected at any 1 time, with an average adult blood volume of 69 to 75 mL/kg of body weight.[4,15,16]

MORPHOLOGY AND NUMBERS OF PERIPHERAL BLOOD CELLS
Erythrocytes

Guinea pig erythrocytes appear as biconcave disks when stained with modified Wright stain (**Fig. 2**). Females have slightly fewer erythrocytes than males. Guinea pig erythrocytes, with a mean cell volume of 84 fL, are larger than erythrocytes in other common laboratory animal species.[17] Anisocytosis is moderate, with width ranging

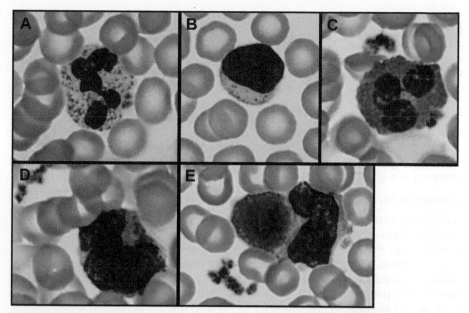

Fig. 2. Representative guinea pig blood cells. (*A*) Heterophil and red blood cells (RBCs). (*B*) Lymphocyte and RBCs. (*C*) Eosinophil, platelets, and RBCs. (*D*) Monocyte, platelets, and RBCs. (*E*) Kurloff cell, platelets, and RBCs. (Wright-Giemsa stain, original magnification 1000x).

between 6.6 and 7.9 μm. An increase in the relative numbers of polychromatophils in the blood smear indicates a regenerative response to anemia. In normal nonanemic cavies, polychromatic erythrocytes may total 25% of circulating erythrocytes in neonates, 4.5% in juveniles, and 1.5% in adults.[17–20] Comparative values of erythrocyte numbers are provided in **Table 2**.

Table 2
Reference ranges of normal hematological parameters in the guinea pig (*Cavia porcellus*)

	Adult Male	Adult Female	Age 2–90 d
RBC ($\times 10^6$/μL)	4.36–6.84	3.35–6.15	4.06–6.02
PCV (%)	37–47	40.9–49.9	33.8–48.8
Hgb (g/dL)	11.6–17.2	11.4–17.0	10.13–15.1
MCV (fL)	71–83	86.1–95.9	77.5–88.7
MCH (pg)	24.2–27.2	23.1–26.3	—
MCHC (%)	29.7–38.9	28.2–34.4	28.3–32.4
Platelets ($\times 10^3$/μL)	260–740	266–634	—
WBC ($\times 10^9$/μL)	5.5–17.5	5.2–16.4	2.66–10.1
Neutrophils (%)	28–56	20.3–41.9	14.8–42.6
Lymphocytes (%)	40.0–62.5	46.4–80.4	52.6–83.2
Eosinophils (%)	1–7	0–7	0.1–3.6
Basophils (%)	0–1.7	0–0.8	0–0.58
Monocytes (%)	3.3–5.3	1.0–2.6	0–3.7

Abbreviations: Hgb, Hemoglobin; MCH, Mean corpuscular hemoglobin; MCHC, Mean corpuscular hemoglobin concentration; MCV, Mean cell volume; PCV, Packed cell volume; RBC, Red blood cell; WBC, white blood cell.
Data from Refs.[13,25,32]

Thrombocytes (Platelets)

In blood smears, guinea pig platelets appear as irregular oval cytoplasmic fragments 2 to 3 μm in diameter with concentric dark inner and lighter outer staining regions (see **Fig. 2**). Reported normal platelet numbers range from 120 to 850/mm³.[2–4,8,13,16,19,21–26] Comparative values of thrombocyte numbers are provided in **Table 2**.

Leukocytes (White Blood Cells)

A variety of factors can influence white blood cell (WBC) total count and differential counts: circadian rhythm (time of day the sample is collected), time of last feeding, breed, and gender.[25] The ranges of total WBC numbers and the WBC cell types observed in a standard differential count are provided in **Table 2**.

Neutrophils (Heterophils)

Guinea pigs heterophils or pseudoeosinophils are the functional counterparts of neutrophils seen in other species and are the next most commonly noted white cell type (see **Fig. 2A**).[8,19] These cells measure 10 to 12 μm in width, with dense nuclei with 5 or more segments. Cytoplasm of heterophils contains multiple pale round eosinophilic inclusions versus the more elongated inclusions seen in eosinophils. Toxicity (accelerated marrow production and shortened maturation time) manifests, as seen in other small animal species, by the presence of increased small basophilic Dohle bodies, cytoplasmic basophilia, and occasionally increased cytoplasmic vacuolation.[27] Reduced nuclear segmentation (bands, left shift) typically accompanies these toxic changes and in most cases can be viewed as markers for the presence of inflammation. Comparative values of neutrophils observed in differential counts in normal guinea pigs are provided in **Table 2**.

Lymphocytes

Lymphocytes are the predominant WBC type in guinea pig blood.[3,4,8,13,16,21,27] Both small and large forms of lymphoid cells are seen, but most are small cells (see **Fig. 2B**).[2,8,13,19] The larger forms can be double the size of the small cells (about the same size as erythrocytes), and may contain a few azurophilic cytoplasmic granules. Comparative values of lymphocytes observed in differential counts in normal guinea pigs are provided in **Table 2**.

Eosinophils

The granules in eosinophils are more pointed than those in heterophils, and they stain more prominently. Eosinophils are larger (10–15 μm wide) with less nuclear segmentation (see **Fig. 2C**).[8,13,17,19] Comparative values of eosinophils observed in differential counts in normal guinea pigs are provided in **Table 2**.

Basophils

Basophils are slightly larger than heterophils with lobulated nuclei and many round variably sized reddish purple to black cytoplasm granules. Comparative values of basophils observed in differential counts in normal guinea pigs are provided in **Table 2**.

Monocytes

Guinea pig monocytes are morphologically similar to those seen in common domestic species, being larger and having darker grey-blue cytoplasm compared with the previously mentioned large lymphocytes (see **Fig. 2D**). Their nuclei tend to be oval to ameboid with a loose lacy chromatin pattern. Comparative values of monocytes observed in differential counts in normal guinea pigs are provided in **Table 2**.

Kurloff Cells

Kurloff cells are a leukocyte type observed in guinea pigs and capybaras (a close relative). The cell is considered a normal incidental feature, appearing as larger mononuclear cells, possibly of lymphoid origin, containing a single reticulated eosinophilic cytoplasmic inclusion 1 to 8 μm wide and present in 3% to 4% of the lymphoid cells or 1% to 2% of the total leukocytes (see **Fig. 2**E).[2] These inclusions consist of a mucopolysaccharide that is toluidine blue, periodic acid-Schiff, and Lendrum stain positive.[2,17] The exact origin and function of these cells is unknown, although it has been speculated that they may function as natural killer cells in the general circulation or as protectors of fetal antigen in the placenta because their numbers can increase under the influence of increased estrogens.[8,13,17,19,28–31]

REFERENCES

1. American Veterinary Medical Association. 2012 U.S. pet ownership & demographic sourcebook. Schaumburg (IL): Membership & Field Services, American Veterinary Medical Association; 2012.
2. Percy DH, Barthold SW. Pathology of laboratory rodents and rabbits. 3rd edition. Ames (IA): Blackwell Pub; 2007. p. 325.
3. Vanderlip SL. The guinea pig handbook. Hauppauge (NY): Barron's; 2003.
4. Harkness JE, Turner PV, VandeWoude S, et al. Harkness and Wagner's biology and medicine of rabbits and rodents. 5th edition. Ames (IA): Wiley-Blackwell; 2010. p. 111.
5. Hawk CT, Leary S. Formulary for laboratory animals. 3rd edition. St Louis (MO): Wiley-Blackwell; 2005.
6. Mitchell MA, Tully TN. Manual of exotic pet practice. St Louis (MO): Saunders Elsevier; 2009. p. 470.
7. Gaertner DJ, Hallman TM, Hankenson FC, et al. Anesthesia and analgesia for laboratory rodents. In: Fish RE, Brown MJ, Danneman PJ, et al, editors. Anesthesia and analgesia in laboratory animals. 2nd edition. San Diego (CA): Academic Press; 2008. p. 279–80.
8. Marshall KL. Clinical hematology of rodent species. Vet Clin North Am Exot Anim Pract 2008;11:523–33.
9. Ott Joslin J. Blood collection techniques in exotic small mammals. J Exot Pet Med 2009;18:117–39.
10. Reuter RE. Venipuncture in the guinea pig. Lab Anim Sci 1987;37:245–6.
11. Hem A, Smith AJ, Solberg P. Saphenous vein puncture for blood sampling of the mouse, rat, hamster, gerbil, guinea pig, ferret and mink. Lab Anim 1998;32:364–8.
12. Dolence D, Jones HE. Pericutaneous phlebotomy and intravenous injection in the guinea pig. Lab Anim Sci 1975;25(1):106–7.
13. Zimmerman LK, Moore MD, Smith SA. Hematology of the guinea pig. In: Weiss DJ, Wardrop KJ, Schalm OW, editors. Schalm's veterinary hematology. 6th edition. Ames (IA): Wiley-Blackwell; 2010. p. 893–8.
14. Hillyer EV, Quesenberry KE. Biology, husbandry, and clinical techniques (of guinea pigs and chinchillas). In: Ferrets, rabbits, and rodents: clinical medicine and surgery. Philadelphia: WB Saunders; 1997. p. 432.
15. Osmond DG, Everett NB. Bone marrow blood volume and total red cell mass of the guinea-pig as determined by 59-Fe-erythrocyte dilution and liquid nitrogen freezing. Q J Exp Physiol Cogn Med Sci 1965;50:1–14.
16. Quesenberry KE, Carpenter JW. Ferrets, rabbits, and rodents: clinical medicine and surgery. 3rd edition. St Louis (MO): Elsevier/Saunders; 2012.

17. Thrall MA. Veterinary hematology and clinical chemistry. 2nd edition. Ames (IA): Wiley-Blackwell; 2012.
18. Albritton EC, American Institute of Biological Sciences, Committee on the Handbook of Biological Data. Standard values in blood, being the first part of a handbook of biological data. Dayton (OH): Air Force, Wright Air Development Center; 1951.
19. Campbell TW, Ellis C. Avian and exotic animal hematology and cytology. 3rd edition. Ames (IA): Blackwell Pub; 2007.
20. Schermer S. The blood morphology of laboratory animals. 3rd edition. Philadelphia: FA Davis; 1967.
21. Suckow MA, Stevens KA, Wilson RP. The laboratory rabbit, guinea pig, hamster, and other rodents. 1st edition. London; Waltham (MA): Academic Press/Elsevier; 2012.
22. Johnson-Delaney CA. Exotic companion medicine handbook for veterinarians. Lake Worth (FL): Wingers Pub; 1995.
23. Kaspareit J, Messow C, Edel J. Blood coagulation studies in guinea pigs (*Cavia porcellus*). Lab Anim 1988;22:206–11.
24. Jones TC, Garner FM, Benirschke K, et al. Pathology of laboratory animals. New York: Springer-Verlag; 1978.
25. Mitruka BM, Rawnsley HM. Clinical biochemical and hematological reference values in normal experimental animals. New York: Masson Pub. USA; 1977.
26. Valenciano CA, Decker SL, Cowell LR. Interpretation of feline leukocyte responses. In: Weiss DJ, Wardrop KJ, Schalm OW, editors. Schalm's veterinary hematology. 6th edition. Ames (IA): Wiley-Blackwell; 2010. p. 335–43.
27. Banks RE. Guinea pig. Exotic small mammal care and husbandry. Ames (IA): Wiley-Blackwell; 2010. p. 115–24.
28. Izard J, Barrellier MT, Quillec M. The Kurloff cell. Its differentiation in the blood and lymphatic system. Cell Tissue Res 1976;173:237–59.
29. Eremin O, Wilson AB, Coombs RR, et al. Antibody-dependent cellular cytotoxicity in the guinea pig: the role of the Kurloff cell. Cell Immunol 1980;55:312–27.
30. Debout C, Quillec M, Izard J. New data on the cytolytic effects of natural killer cells (Kurloff cells) on a leukemic cell line (guinea pig L2C). Leuk Res 1999;23: 137–47.
31. Marshall AH, Swettenham KV, Vernon-Roberts B, et al. Studies on the function of the Kurloff cell. Int Arch Allergy Appl Immunol 1971;40:137–52.
32. Jain NC. Normal values in blood of laboratory, furbearing and miscellaneous zoo, domestic and wild animals. In: Jain NC, editor. Schalm's veterinary hematology. Philadelphia: Lea & Febiger; 1986. p. 274–343.

Hematology of Camelids

Linda Vap, DVM, DACVP*, Andrea A. Bohn, DVM, PhD, DACVP

KEYWORDS

- Llama • Alpaca • Analyzer • Quality assurance

KEY POINTS

- Hematology between new and old world camels is similar.
- Leukocyte morphology is similar to other food and fiber animals.
- Camelid erythrocyte morphology differs from other mammals.
- Automated instruments may produce erroneous erythron results as a result of unique camelid erythrocyte morphology.

Mammals falling in to the family of Camelidae have been categorized as the true camels (dromedary, one-humped and Bactrian, 2-humped), new world camels (NWC, llama and alpaca), and South American camels (guanaco and vicuña). A North American veterinarian is most likely to come across llamas and alpacas owing to their use as a source of food, fiber, labor, and companionship. An exotic animal veterinarian may be required to evaluate any of the camel-like animals because zoos exhibit a wide variety of animals from around the world. Fortunately, much of their hematology is similar to that of other mammals. The primary issue with camelid hematology is related to the fact that some instruments are not suitable for analyzing their small, numerous, elliptical erythrocytes. The following provides an overview of normal and abnormal findings in camelid blood as well as how to ensure accurate results from automated methods.

NORMAL HEMATOLOGY
Normal Morphology

With basic hematology skills and a reliable staining method, neutrophils, lymphocytes, monocytes, and eosinophils should be readily recognizable during microscopic examination for a manual differential count. Microscopic examination allows for the evaluation of morphologic changes and the presence of other cells not typically detected by instruments, such as band neutrophils, immature lymphocytes, and others. Small, intermediate, and large lymphocytes may be observed.[1] Eosinophils may normally have hyposegmented nuclei (Fig. 1), and one might note a relatively high proportion of granulated lymphocytes in healthy animals when performing manual differentials.[2] The granules will be most noticeable when alcohol-based Romanowsky stains are used rather than quick stains that are aqueous based.[3]

Department of Microbiology, Immunology, and Pathology, College of Veterinary Medicine and Biomedical Sciences, Colorado State University, Fort Collins, CO 80523-1610, USA
* Corresponding author.
E-mail address: Linda.Vap@colostate.edu

Vet Clin Exot Anim 18 (2015) 41–49
http://dx.doi.org/10.1016/j.cvex.2014.09.010
1094-9194/15/$ – see front matter © 2015 Elsevier Inc. All rights reserved.

Platelets tend to be smaller and may be more numerous than many species. Because of their small size, some automated analyzers may ignore some platelets as debris and report erroneously low results. If this is the case, a semiquantitative (eg, low or adequate) estimate from the blood film can be substituted. As with any species, examining the film for platelet clumping is prudent when assessing suspected low platelet concentrations.

Camelids vary from other mammals in their erythrocyte morphology. Rather than the typical biconcave disc observed in most mammals, normal camelid erythrocytes are oval, flat, and lack central pallor. The flat contour lends them to a folding artifact (**Fig. 2**) that may concern the inexperienced observer. A few erythrocytes may contain rhomboid or hexagonal hemoglobin crystals, an intriguing but idiopathic and apparently nonpathogenic phenomenon.[2] Camelid erythrocytes are also smaller in volume and significantly more numerous than most mammalian erythrocytes, with an upper limit of normal that approaches 18 million/uL.[4]

Camelid blood contains less than 1 reticulocyte per 1000× field in health. When at altitudes of 14,000 ft, higher erythrocyte turnover may be reflected by reticulocytes composing up to 1.5% of the population.[5] These younger cells are larger and plumper than mature cells and polychromatophilic with Romanowsky-type stains (see **Fig. 2**). Nucleated erythrocytes are observed in low numbers in healthy animals. These erythrocytes will appear more rounded and contain a dense, round nucleus. The cytoplasm may be polychromatophilic. Manual reticulocyte counts can be performed on fresh whole blood with a supravital stain as new methylene blue or brilliant cresyl blue stain (**Fig. 3**). This method is tedious and requires an accurate erythrocyte count in order to calculate absolute numbers of reticulocytes.

Reference Intervals

Previously published reference intervals for erythrocyte data are problematic, especially for camels. Data are incomplete or only relative numbers (%) of leukocytes were often reported.[6,7] In addition, methods for determining ranges are often not described; when one critically evaluates the reported reference intervals, it can easily be deduced that errors were made because the ranges are often very broad, especially regarding the mean cell volume (MCV) and mean corpuscular hemoglobin

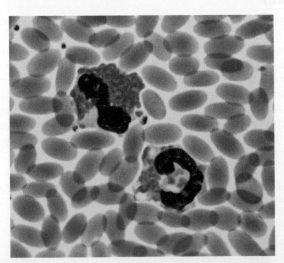

Fig. 1. Banded eosinophils (Wright-Giemsa, original magnification 1000×).

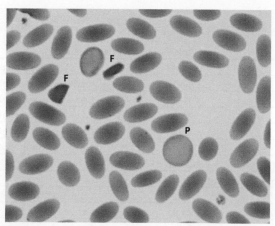

Fig. 2. Normal erythrocyte morphology exhibiting flat, elliptical cells, no central pallor, and cell folding (F). One polychromatophilic erythrocyte is visible (P). Platelets are small and granular. Camel (Wright-Giemsa, original magnification 1000×).

concentration (MCHC). These parameters should be fairly consistent within a species. It is presumed that the small size, high numbers, and elliptical shape of the camelid erythrocyte contributed to these errors. In general, there can be rather large inherent errors when counting erythrocytes using the hemocytometer method. Particle counters can be more accurate, but red blood cell (RBC) concentrations will be incorrect if improper threshold settings or insufficient dilutions are used. If all of the erythrocytes are not counted, the RBC concentration obtained is falsely low; this will also cause errors in the red cell indices calculated from this value.[2]

Table 1 provides approximate normal values for adult llamas after eliminating obviously erroneous information and combining data from several remaining sources.[2,8]

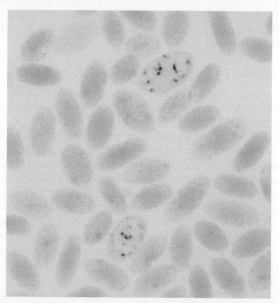

Fig. 3. Reticulocytes (brilliant cresyl blue, original magnification 1000×).

Table 1
Approximate reference intervals for adult llamas

CBC Parameter	Reference Intervals	Comment
PCV (%)	27–45	Camels possibly slightly lower
RBC ($\times 10^6$/uL)	10–17	Camels possibly slightly lower
Hgb (g/dL)	11–19	Camels possibly slightly lower
MCV (fL)	21–31	Camels possibly slightly broader
MCHC (g/dL)	39–48	Camels possibly slightly lower
WBC ($\times 10^3$/uL)	7.5–22	Camels possibly slightly lower
Band neutrophils ($\times 10^3$/uL)	0–0.4	—
Segmented neutrophils ($\times 10^3$/uL)	4.6–16.0	—
Lymphocytes ($\times 10^3$/uL)	1–10	Up to 30% granulated
Monocytes ($\times 10^3$/uL)	<1.0	—
Eosinophils ($\times 10^3$/uL)	0–5	Tend to have hyposegmented nuclei
Basophils ($\times 10^3$/uL)	<1.0	—
Platelets ($\times 10^3$/uL)	150–800	—
Reticulocytes ($\times 10^3$/uL; %)	12–79,000; 0–0.6	0–3 Nucleated RBC/100 WBC

Abbreviations: CBC, complete blood count; Hgb, hemoglobin; PCV, packed-cell volume; WBC, white blood cell count.
Adapted from Refs.[2,4,8]

The resulting ranges remain rather broad presumably due to differences in methodology as well as husbandry and environmental conditions. Reference intervals for leukocyte differential results are reported here in absolute numbers since interpreting only relative (%) results can be misleading. Reference intervals for alpacas using an impedance analyzer[9] and a laser-based hematology analyzer have been published.[10] Using or establishing reference intervals specific for the methods used and representative of the patient population is recommended when dealing with camelid herds on a regular basis. Obtaining baseline values from samples collected during health to compare to the same animal when sick is an alternative when dealing with low numbers of individual animals.

ABNORMAL HEMATOLOGY
Leukon

When evaluating the leukon, primary differentials include excitement, stress, inflammation, and neoplasia (leukemia). The main reason for recognizing excitement or stress responses is so that inflammation is not overdiagnosed. Younger animals may have higher lymphocyte counts than their adult counterparts.[9,11] As with other mammals, a mature neutrophilia and lymphopenia is consistent with stress; eosinopenia may also be noted. Inflammation is typically characterized by neutrophilia with a left shift. Toxic changes within neutrophils, such as Döhle bodies, reflect rapid marrow turnover and may also be present. Hyperfibrinogenemia may accompany the microscopic findings. It is important to note that the inflammatory response is a dynamic process; if the inflammatory stimulus overwhelms the marrow, low or normal leukocyte counts may result. Alternatively, the marrow may fully compensate under chronic inflammatory stimuli and produce only a mature neutrophilia. Stress and inflammation can occur simultaneously.

Lymphoma has been reported with some frequency in camelids; however, leukemia has only rarely been reported.[12–15] Leukemia should be suspected if a high leukocyte count is obtained, unless the cells are predominantly composed of mature and band neutrophils or it is associated with only a modest increase in the number of small lymphocytes in a young animal. Blood films should be evaluated to microscopically confirm which cells are present, and it is often best to confirm leukemia by sending the blood and bone marrow samples along with freshly prepared films to a clinical pathologist for evaluation.

Erythron

As in all species, anemia can result from blood loss, erythrocyte destruction, or decreased production of erythrocytes from the bone marrow. Regenerative anemia is typically associated with blood loss or hemolysis. Nonregenerative anemia is most commonly associated with anemia of chronic disease, which results in decreased erythropoiesis.

Hypochromic anemia with or without evidence of regeneration and accompanying macrocytosis may be observed in cases of iron deficiency, chronic inflammation, endoparasitism and ectoparasitism, and copper deficiency.[11,16] Chronic iron deficiency may be associated with microcytosis and increased numbers of folded cells.[16] Morphologic erythrocyte irregularities, such as dacryocytes (teardrop-shaped cells), spindloid cells, and irregular hemoglobin distribution, may be observed with iron deficiency and marked anemia with other pathogeneses (**Fig. 4**).[16,17] Maple leaf toxicity resulting in Heinz body–related hemolytic anemia has been reported.[18] Heinz bodies consist of denatured hemoglobin. These pale, rounded inclusions observed with Romanowsky stains will be a more apparent teal blue color with reticulocyte stains.

Mycoplasma haemolamae (previously known as *Eperythrozoon*) is a hemotropic, wall-less bacteria observed in the blood of NWC.[19–21] This organism is visible under high-resolution light microscopy as a small rod or circular structure on the erythrocyte surface (**Fig. 5**). It will fall off the cells a few hours after collection, so examination of freshly prepared films is crucial. It is possible that the number of circulating organisms is too low for observation, that organisms are sequestered elsewhere in the body, or that they are confused with stain precipitate. Suspect cases can be confirmed by

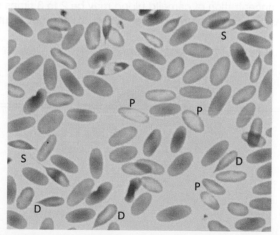

Fig. 4. Blood from an NWC with iron deficiency. Note dacryocytes (D), spindloid cells (S), and cells with increased central pallor (P) (Wright-Giemsa, original magnification 1000×).

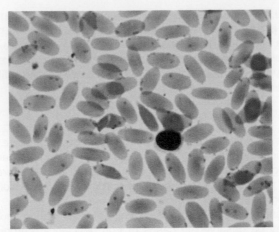

Fig. 5. Erythrocytes from an NWC cria with surface-associated *M haemolamae* organisms and one nRBC. Some organisms are free in the background (Wright-Giemsa, original magnification 1000×).

polymerase chain reaction (PCR). Regenerative responses, with (**Fig. 6**) or without agglutination, are expected with infectious anemia but can also be observed with idiopathic immune-mediated hemolytic anemia.

Relative polycythemia is expected with dehydration and is a common sequela to diarrhea. Aside from dehydration, polycythemia has been reported in 2 case reports. One case was idiopathic and one was associated with a granulosa theca cell tumor.[22,23]

METHODOLOGY

It is important that data obtained for the evaluation of animals' health are reliable. The following information and guidelines are included to help you determine the feasibility of using your in-house hematology analyzer for camelid samples.

In-house hematology analyzers fall into 2 basic technology types: impedance (electrical sizing as cells pass through an aperture) and flow cytometry (laser light scatter). The erythrocyte concentration of camelid blood may be 2 to 3 times that of common domestic species. If samples from these species are not diluted sufficiently,

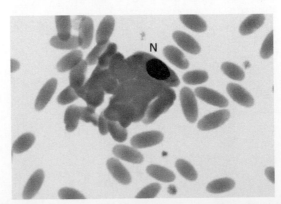

Fig. 6. Erythrocytes exhibiting autoagglutination and one nRBC. This alpaca was previously diagnosed with *M haemolamae* (Wright-Giemsa, original magnification 1000×).

coincidence may occur where cells pass through the aperture or in front of the laser in pairs rather than singly. As a result, 2 small cells passing through the measuring device are counted as one large cell. In addition, sizing thresholds may not be set sufficiently low enough to capture the smallest cells of the erythrocyte population. The outcome is that the instrument may report erroneously low erythrocyte counts with an accurate hemoglobin concentration, resulting in a falsely increased MCHC. High MCHC values are not physiologically possible and support instrument error once hemolysis and lipemia in the sample are ruled out.

Absolute differential counts require a total white blood cell count (WBC) or nucleated cell count (NCC) and a differential count. An NCC includes nucleated erythrocytes (nRBCs), and most automated instruments include nRBCs when counting leukocytes. When this is the case, the nRBCs can be included as a distinct cell type during the manual differential count; absolute concentrations are then derived for each of the nucleated cells. In-house instruments are fairly reliable for obtaining NCCs; their use is preferred over manual methods for accuracy, precision, and reduced technical time. Similar to other mammalian leukocytes, camelid neutrophils and, somewhat less so, lymphocytes can be reliably counted by in-house instruments. Eosinophil concentrations tend to run higher in camelids than many mammals; when sufficiently high enough, they may also be accurately counted by automated methods. As a general rule of thumb, monocytes and basophils are present in proportions too low to be accurately measured; but this variability is rarely clinical significant.[10] A quick scan of a blood film can assess whether automated differentials appear reasonable.

It behooves the veterinarian to ensure he or she is interpreting accurate results, which can be done by ensuring technical staff members are following 3 simple quality-assurance procedures[24]:

- Ensure results of a manual packed-cell volume (PCV) agree within 2% to 3% of the automated hematocrit (Hct) value obtained from the analyzer on the same well-mixed sample.
- Ensure results obtained from running commercial quality control material (QCM) are within expected ranges.
  - Even though the QCM will represent blood from mammals other than camelids, evaluating results from it is a highly recommended routine process when using automated methods.
- Ensure the MCHC is at or less than the upper limit of normal, up to approximately 36 g/dL for domestic mammals and up to approximately 49 g/dL for camelids.
  - The presence of either hemolysis or lipemia erroneously increases the MCHC value. Examining the supernatant after spinning a microhematocrit tube to obtain the PCV can easily check samples. If hemolysis and/or lipemia are observed, ignore the MCHC result from this sample and test a sample from another animal.

If the criteria are met for the aforementioned steps, the instrument is probably running appropriately. If the results obtained from the QCM are within the expected limits but the PCV and Hct do not match and/or the MCHC is high only on camelid samples, the instrument may be running as it should, but it is not capable of accurately measuring camelid erythrocytes. If this is the case, the hemoglobin concentration is the only erythrocyte-related information that can be used from the instrument. A manual PCV can replace the automated Hct and the MCHC can be calculated (10 × Hgb/PCV, where *Hgb* is hemoglobin). The MCV is a calculation that requires a manual erythrocyte count, a time-consuming process that is generally not recommended, as it fails to provide sufficient additional information. If the MCHC is running high on both camelid and noncamelid samples, the instrument is probably malfunctioning.

REFERENCES

1. Azwai SM, Abdouslam OE, Al-Bassam LS, et al. Morphological characteristics of blood cells in clinically normal adult llamas (Lama glama). Veterinarski Arhiv 2007;77:69–79.
2. Houten Van, Weiser MG, Johnson L, et al. Reference hematologic values and morphologic features of blood cells in healthy adult llamas. Am J Vet Res 1992;53(10):1773–5.
3. Allison RW, Velguth KE. Appearance of granulated cells on blood films stained by automated aqueous versus methanolic Romanowsky methods. Vet Clin Pathol 2010;39(1):99–104.
4. Weiser MG, Fettman MJ, Van Houten DS, et al. Characterization of erythrocytic indices and serum iron values in healthy llamas. Am J Vet Res 1992;53:1776–9.
5. Reynafarje C, Faura J, Paredes A, et al. Erythrokinetics in high-altitude-adapted animals (llama, alpaca, and vicuña). J Appl Physiol 1968;24(1):93–7.
6. Alhadrami GA. Comparative haematology in the camel calf and adult racing camel (Camelus dromedarius). In: Gahlot TK, editor. Selected research on camelid physiology and nutrition. Bikaner (India): The Camelid Publishers; 2004. p. 378–9 (taken from Journal of Camel Practice and Research 1997;4(1):13).
7. Nyang'ao JM, Olaho-Mukani W, Maribei JM, et al. A study of some haematological and biochemical parameters of the normal dromedary camel in Kenya. In: Gahlot TK, editor. Selected research on camelid physiology and nutrition. Bikaner (India): The Camelid Publishers; 2004. p. 380–4 (taken from Journal of Camel Practice and Research 1997;4(1):31-33).
8. Fowler ME, Zinkl JG. Reference ranges for hematologic and serum biochemical values in llamas (Lama glama). Am J Vet Res 1989;50(12):2049–53.
9. Hajduk P. Haematological reference values for alpacas. Aust Vet J 1992;69: 89–90.
10. Dawson DR, DeFrancisco RJ, Stokol T. Reference intervals for hematologic and coagulation tests in adult alpacas (Vicugna pacos). Vet Clin Pathol 2011;40: 504–12.
11. Hawkey CM, Gullan FM. Haematology of clinically normal and abnormal captive llamas and guanacos. Vet Rec 1988;122:232–4.
12. Cebra CK, Garry FB, Powers BE, et al. Lymphosarcoma in 10 new world camelids. J Vet Intern Med 1995;9:381–5.
13. Valentine BA, Martin JM. Prevalence of neoplasia in llamas and alpacas (Oregon State University, 2001-2006). J Vet Diagn Invest 2007;19:202–4.
14. Steinberg JD, Olver CS, Davis WC, et al. Acute myeloid leukemia with multilineage dysplasia in an alpaca. Vet Clin Pathol 2008;37:289–97.
15. Martin JM, Valentine BA, Cebra CK, et al. Malignant round cell neoplasia in llamas and alpacas. Vet Pathol 2009;46:288–98.
16. Morin DE, Garry FB, Weiser MG, et al. Hematologic features of iron deficiency anemia in llamas. Vet Pathol 1992;29(5):400–4.
17. Tornquist SJ. Hematology of camelids. In: Weiss DJ, Wardrop KJ, editors. Schalm's veterinary hematology. 6th edition. Ames (IA): Blackwell Publishing Ltd; 2010. p. 910–7.

18. Dewitt SF, Bedenice D, Mazan MR. Hemolysis and Heinz body formation associated with ingestion of red maple leaves in two alpacas. J Am Vet Med Assoc 2004;225(4):578–83, 539.
19. McLaughlin BG, Evans CN, McLaughlin PS, et al. An Eperythrozoon-like parasite in llamas. J Am Vet Med Assoc 1990;197:1170–5.
20. Reagan WJ, Garry F, Thrall MA, et al. The clinicopathologic, light, and scanning electron microscopic features of eperythrozoonosis in four naturally-infected llamas. Vet Pathol 1990;27:426–31.
21. Messick JB, Walker PG, Raphael W, et al. 'Candidatus Mycoplasma haemodidelphidis' sp. nov., 'Candidatus Mycoplasma haemolamae' sp. nov. and *Mycoplasma haemocanis* comb. nov., haemotrophic parasites from a naturally infected opossum (*Didelphis virginiana*), alpaca (*Lama pacos*) and dog (*Canis familiaris*): phylogenetic and secondary structural relatedness of their 16S rRNA genes to other mycoplasmas. Int J Syst Evol Microbiol 2002;52:693–8.
22. Anderson DE, Couto CG, Oglesbee M. Granulosa theca cell tumor with erythrocytosis in a llama. Can Vet J 2010;51(10):1157–60.
23. Gentz EJ, Pearson EG, Lassen ED, et al. Polycythemia in a llama. J Am Vet Med Assoc 1994;204(9):1490–2.
24. Vap LM, Harr K, Friedrichs KR, et al. ASVCP quality assurance guidelines: control of preanalytical, analytical and postanalytical factors in veterinary laboratories related to hematology for mammalian and non-mammalian species, hemostasis, and crossmatching. Vet Clin Pathol 2012;41(1):8–17.

Avian Hematology

Michael P. Jones, DVM, DABVP (Avian)

KEYWORDS

- Avian hematology • Erythrocyte • Leukocyte • Anemia • Leukocytosis • Leukopenia

KEY POINTS

- Hematology is an invaluable part of the clinical management of avian patients.
- The half-life of avian erythrocytes is shorter than mammalian erythrocytes.
- Acute blood loss is the most common cause of regenerative anemia in birds.
- Nonregenerative anemia is the most common type of anemia described in birds.
- The heterophil is the most common granulocyte found in the peripheral blood of birds.
- Lymphocytes are second to heterophils in frequency in most avian species except Amazon parrots and canaries, in which the lymphocytes may be the predominate leukocytes and may account for up to 70% of circulating leukocytes.

AVIAN HEMATOLOGY

Hematology is an invaluable part of the clinical management of avian patients. To evaluate the health of their patients, the clinical progression of disease, and response to therapy, avian veterinarians should be well versed in sample collection, cellular identification, and interpretation of results of the hemogram. Avian erythrocytes and leukocytes may be evaluated with automated or manual techniques. Packed cell volume (PCV), total erythrocyte count, hemoglobin concentration, Wintrobe indices, reticulocyte count, erythrocyte morphology, total white blood cell (WBC) count, and leukocyte differentials are all used to evaluate the avian hemogram. It should be noted that although hematologic reference intervals and ranges have been established for many avian species, determined values may vary by age, sex, season/environment, and hormonal influences.[1–4] In one study, PCV and total erythrocyte count tended to be higher in male birds compared with female birds, and also increased with age. In another study,[5] only the erythrocyte count tended to increase significantly with age in bald eagles.

The reader should know that although an understanding of avian hematologic techniques is essential, methods of sample collection, processing, and analysis of blood samples are elaborated in detail elsewhere.[1,6–8]

The author has nothing to disclose.

Department of Small Animal Clinical Sciences, College of Veterinary Medicine, University of Tennessee, 2407 River Drive, Room C247, Knoxville, TN 37996, USA

E-mail address: mpjones@utk.edu

Vet Clin Exot Anim 18 (2015) 51–61
http://dx.doi.org/10.1016/j.cvex.2014.09.012
1094-9194/15/$ – see front matter © 2015 Elsevier Inc. All rights reserved.

AVIAN ERYTHROCYTE MORPHOLOGY

Avian erythrocytes are oval or elliptical in shape with a central, oval nucleus and are mostly uniform in appearance among avian species (**Fig. 1**). Comparatively, they are larger than mammalian erythrocytes. When stained with Wright or Romanowsky stains, healthy, mature erythrocytes have an orange-pink–colored cytoplasm. The nucleus, which is uniformly clumped in appearance, stains a dark purple color and becomes more condensed with age.[1,3]

Polychromatophilic Erythrocytes and Reticulocytes

The half-life of avian erythrocytes is relatively short (28–45 days), which results in the regular appearance of polychromatophilic erythrocytes (approximately 1%–5% of the total erythrocyte count) in the circulating blood pool.[9] These polychromatic erythrocytes are more rounded in appearance, their cytoplasm stains more basophilic, and their nuclei are more rounded with less densely packed chromatin when compared with mature erythrocytes. They, along with reticulocytes, are indicative of bone marrow activity and erythrocyte regenerative capacity in avian species.[1,3] Polychromatophilic erythrocytes appear as reticulocytes when stained with Wright or new methylene blue stains. However, a significant number of avian erythrocytes contain basophilic granular material when supravitally stained; therefore, reticulocytes are defined as having a distinct ring of reticular material (characteristic clumps of residual cytoplasmic RNA) partially or completely encircling the nucleus.[3,9,10] Although the percentages of polychromatophils parallel the percentage of reticulocytes, the reticulocyte percentage is a more precise measurement of erythrocyte regeneration.[11] Immature erythrocytes with basophilic staining cytoplasm and a smaller, more rounded appearance than mature red blood cells are most commonly rubricytes.[1,3] They are an indication of a marked regenerative response in avian patients.

Anisocytosis

Variation in size and of avian erythrocytes is occasionally seen in peripheral blood smears.[1] Slight anisocytosis is considered an insignificant finding in birds.[3] Automated methods of performing erythrocyte counts can calculate the degree of anisocytosis using the red cell distribution width (RDW%), which measures variation in red blood cell size, or mean corpuscular volume.[7] RDW% may vary depending on the patient's age or even between laboratories. Normal psittacine RDW% is 10% to 11%. Percentages above those indicate an increase in anisocytosis.[7]

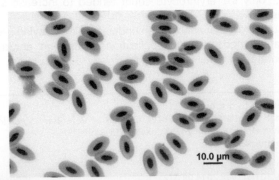

Fig. 1. Erythrocytes in the blood film of a hawk (*Buteo jamaicensis*) (Wright-Giemsa stain).

Poikilocytes

Erythrocytes that exhibit variations in shape are termed poikilocytes. These cells are more susceptible to damage, and as a result, have a shorter half-life than other erythrocytes. These may appear round, elongated, or irregular. The erythrocyte nucleus also may vary in appearance, location, and number, or on rare occasions may be absent.[7,12] Erythrocytes that are anucleated are termed erythroplastids.[8] Erythrocytes, which appear round with oval nuclei, are indicative of asynchronous maturation associated with accelerated erythropoiesis.[1,9] Binucleate erythrocytes, which indicate abnormal erythropoiesis, are often associated with severe, chronic inflammatory or neoplastic processes.[12]

Anemia

Most birds have a PCV between 35% and 55%; however, reference ranges and reference intervals for individual species should be considered. Anemias are usually the result of increased loss or destruction of erythrocytes or decreased production and are demonstrated by a decrease in the total erythrocyte count and PCV. Anemias due to decreased production appear to be mild anemias in contrast to more severe anemias caused by disease processes that affect the peripheral blood or bone marrow. Anemias are classified as regenerative, nonregenerative, hemolytic, or hemorrhagic.

Regenerative anemia
Regenerative anemias are characterized by the presence of polychromasia, reticulocytosis, macrocytosis, increased RDW%, and anisocytosis. Acute blood loss is the most common cause of a regenerative anemia in birds.

Nonregenerative anemia
Nonregenerative anemias seem to be the most common type of anemia described in birds, and indicate a lack of appropriate bone marrow response.[7] Etiologies include chronic inflammatory conditions, chronic infectious diseases (tuberculosis, colibacillosis, salmonellosis, aspergillosis), some viral diseases (West Nile virus), acute or chronic chlamydophilosis, and toxicosis (lead or aflatoxicosis), iron deficiency, endocrinopathies (hypothyroidism), and leukemia.[1–3]

Hemolytic anemia
Hemolytic anemias are often regenerative in nature and indicated by increased polychromasia, macrocytosis, anisocytosis, and reticulocytosis. Disorders that may cause a hemolytic anemia include erythrocyte destruction by parasites (*Plasmodium* spp and *Aegyptianella* sp), bacterial septicemia, acute toxicosis (oil ingestion, lead, zinc, petroleum products, and aflatoxicosis) and immune-mediated conditions.[1] However, the latter has not been well documented in birds.[13]

Hemorrhagic anemia
Hemorrhagic anemias result from blood loss due to trauma, gastrointestinal parasitism, coagulation disorders (as in conure bleeding syndrome, rodenticide toxicosis, and aflatoxicosis), organ rupture or ulceration, aneurysms, and some viral diseases. Following acute hemorrhage there is often a rapid increase (in hours) during which erythropoiesis increases dramatically.[1,14]

Polycythemia

Polycythemia is defined as an elevated PCV and erythrocyte count and is considered uncommon in birds.[1,3,7] Polycythemia may be categorized as absolute or relative polycythemia. Relative polycythemia is due to either redistribution of erythrocytes or the result of hemoconcentration or loss of plasma volume as a result of dehydration.[2,8] Birds do not store reserve erythrocytes in their spleen so relative polycythemia due to redistribution of erythrocytes is not seen in birds. Absolute polycythemia is further divided into primary polycythemia (polycythemia vera) or secondary polycythemia. Polycythemia vera is rare in birds[1,3] and is caused by a myeloproliferative disease that results in an increased production of erythrocytes.[3,8] Secondary polycythemia is a response to hypoxia, which results in an increased production of erythropoietin. Disease conditions that lead to secondary polycythemia include chronic pulmonary diseases, cardiac disease, iron storage disease, rickets, renal disease or renal neoplasia, or a physiologic response to high altitude.[3,8] Polycythemia is often a diagnosis of exclusion of possible etiologies. Treatment of polycythemia involves alleviation of the underlying cause and phlebotomy.[3]

Hemoparasites

Hemoparasites are seen in many species of captive and free-ranging birds. The most commonly identified hemoparasites include *Hemoproteus* spp, *Plasmodium* spp, and *Leukocytozoon* spp. Many avian species are susceptible to infection with hemoparasites, although clinical disease seems to be more significant in some species than others. *Hemoproteus* and *Leukocytozoon* may be found in large numbers within the bloodstream with no apparent clinical signs. Both *Hemoproteus* (**Fig. 2**) and *Leukocytozoon* (**Fig. 3**) are generally considered to be of low pathogenicity unless there is concurrent disease. However, once the underlying disease process is treated or alleviated, the presence of these hemoparasites in the blood seems to dissipate. *Hemoproteus* spp are sometimes confused with *Plasmodium* spp when evaluating a blood smear, except that *Hemoproteus* gametocytes tend to encircle more than half of the erythrocyte nucleus without displacing it from its central position and are not found in any other blood cells.[3]

   Plasmodium spp, the causative agent of avian malaria, can be pathogenic in a number of avian species, especially passerines (canaries), waterfowl, birds of prey, penguins, and poultry.[3] Intraerythrocytic gametocytes appear round or elongated and commonly displace the erythrocyte nucleus.[1,3,8] In addition, schizonts (containing merozoites) may be found in erythrocytes, and gametocytes and schizonts can be identified in other blood cells.[3,8] Clinical signs of *Plasmodium* infections include lethargy and depression, anorexia, weight loss, increased respiratory effort, biliverdinuria,

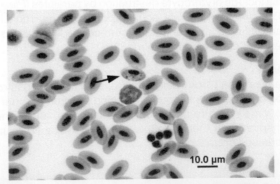

Fig. 2. *Hemoproteus* gametocyte (*arrow*) within an erythrocyte in the blood film of a hawk (*Buteo jamaicensis*) (Wright-Giemsa stain).

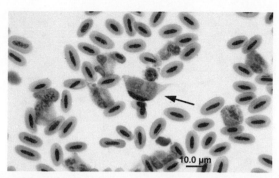

Fig. 3. *Leukocytozoon* gametocyte (*arrow*) in the blood film of a hawk (*Buteo jamaicensis*) (Wright-Giemsa stain).

and acute death. Laboratory diagnostics test results also may reveal hemolytic anemia, leukocytosis, and lymphocytosis.[1,3,8]

AVIAN LEUKOCYTE MORPHOLOGY

Avian leukocytes include granulocytes (heterophils, eosinophils, and basophils), mononuclear cells (lymphocytes and monocytes), and thrombocytes. Total WBC count, estimated WBC count, and leukocyte differential performed by automated or manual techniques are all used to evaluate leukocytes in the avian hemogram. Specific methods of sample collection, processing, and analysis of blood samples are elaborated in detail elsewehere.[1,2,8]

Leukocytosis refers to an elevation of the total WBC count and is most often associated with inflammatory diseases (gout, egg-yolk coelomitis, degenerative joint disease, or allergy), infectious diseases (bacteria, fungi, or parasites), or stress, or may actually be a normal finding in young birds.[2,6–8] When a marked leukocytosis (total WBC >30,000 10^3/μL) is noted, infectious diseases, such as chlamydophila, aspergillosis, mycobacteriosis, pneumonia, coelomitis, salpingitis, coelomitis, toxicosis (lead), neoplasia, and some and viral infections should be strongly considered. Stress leukograms have been reported in macaws, African gray parrots, cockatoos, and ratites, as well as other avian species, and may occur following travel, capture and restraint for physical examination, exercise, and trauma.[6,7,14,15] Although considered rare, excessively high leukocyte counts may indicate leukemia.

Leukopenia is often associated with chronic infectious or inflammatory diseases, severe, overwhelming bacterial or viral infections (circovirus infections in young birds, herpes virus, or polyomavirus), toxicosis, chemotherapeutic agents, or septicemia.[2,6,7] Improper sample handling may cause an artifactual decrease in WBC count due to blood clotting.[2]

Heterophil

The heterophil is the most common granulocyte found in peripheral blood and is usually the most predominant WBC. Avian heterophils contain eosinophilic, oval or spindle shaped granules which tend to cover most of the heterophil's nucleus (**Fig. 4**).[14] The nucleus contains coarsely clumped chromatin and usually has two to three lobes.[1,14]

Heterophilia may be associated with acute or chronic inflammatory and infectious diseases, stress, or may be normal in young birds.[2] In many instances, the severity of the leukocytosis associated with a heterophilia may correlate with the severity of

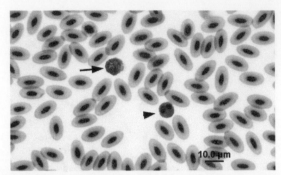

Fig. 4. Heterophil (*arrow*) and eosinophil (*arrowhead*) in the blood film of a hawk (*Buteo jamaicensis*) (Wright-Giemsa stain).

the disease.[10] The differential diagnoses for heterophilia mirror those for leukocytosis. Chlamydophila, aspergillosis, and mycobacteriosis, pneumonia, coelomitis, salpingitis, coelomitis, toxicoses (lead and zinc), neoplasia, and viral infections are all likely causes of a heterophilic inflammatory response.[1,6,7]

True heteropenia is rare in avian patients, but is usually associated with a leukopenia.[15] Overwhelming infectious diseases, bacterial septicemia, and some viral diseases, especially circovirus infections in African gray parrots (*Psittacus erithacus erithacus*), may cause a heteropenia.[1,3,6,7] In some instances, heteropenia occurs when significant numbers of ruptured leukocytes (smudge cells), likely heterophils, are present in a blood smear.[15] In some species, such as canaries and Amazon parrots, lymphocytes may be the predominate leukocyte in the hemogram.

Immature (band) heterophils are rarely seen in peripheral blood smears; however, when present, they may indicate severe, acute inflammation in which the demand for heterophils exceeds their release from the bone marrow.[3] Band heterophils are seen in peripheral blood smears within the first 12 to 24 hours after the onset of inflammatory disease, and are released in response to cytokines and other inflammatory mediators.[1,3,8] A degenerative left shift occurs when the increase in immature heterophils is greater than the number of mature heterophils and is associated with a persistent leukopenia. Left shifts may result from acute chlamydophila infections or other overwhelming diseases (such as mycobacteriosis, systemic fungal disease, septicemia).[1,2,7,15] A degenerative left shift indicates a poor to guarded prognosis. Band heterophils are characterized by an indistinctly lobulated or even horseshoe-shaped nucleus, cytoplasm that stains basophilic, and fewer granules that are round and stain deeply basophilic.[2] Care must be taken not to confuse them with basophils.

Toxic heterophils are a significant finding on an avian blood smear and are seen with severe diseases that affect production and release from the bone marrow.[7] Toxic heterophils have increased cytoplasmic basophilia, vacuolization of the cytoplasm, hypersegmentation and degeneration of the nucleus, degranulation or abnormal granules, and basophilic cytoplasmic inclusions (**Fig. 5**).[1,2,7,14,16]

Eosinophil

The avian eosinophil is a round cell with a pale blue cytoplasm in contrast to the colorless cytoplasm of the heterophil (see **Fig. 4**).[1,7] Typically, avian eosinophil granules are round in shape, although size, shape, and color may vary among species. Eosinophil granules are brighter in color when compared with the heterophil granules. This difference is due to a higher concentration of arginine in the eosinophil granules.[1,7,14]

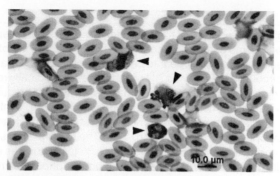

Fig. 5. Toxic heterophils (*arrowheads*) in the blood film of a cormorant (*Phalacrocorax auritus*) (Wright-Giemsa stain).

Eosinophil granules also lack the refractile central body of the heterophil granule.[1,6,7] Eosinophilia is often relative in that there may be an increased percentage of eosinophils but not a change in the absolute value of circulating eosinophils.[7] Etiologies for eosinophilia in birds often can be a mystery. Eosinophilia is rare in many avian species but common in others. When an eosinophilia is present, it may be due to marked tissue damage, parasitic diseases, such as giardiasis, ascaridiasis, and cestodiasis, or allergic conditions, but this is not always the case.[1,3,6,7,12] Eosinopenia is rarely reported in birds.[7]

Basophil

Basophils are also uncommon in peripheral blood smears of avian species; however, when seen, they should not be confused with toxic heterophils (**Fig. 6**). Avian basophils are slightly smaller than heterophils, with clear cytoplasm, a lightly blue stained nucleus that is nonlobed, and round basophilic granules that often obscure the nucleus.[2,3] Very little is known about the avian basophils; they appear to participate in early inflammatory responses and possibly allergic (hypersensitivity) reactions. Basophilia may be observed in birds with respiratory disease or tissue damage, and may be common in active chlamydial infections (particularly in budgerigars and Amazon parrots).[1,3,6,7,16] In Amazon parrots, such as the green-cheeked Amazon parrot (*Amazona viridigenalis*), the basophil granules appear to be larger and more prominent than in other psittacine species.[17] It is common for normal hemograms to not show any basophils.

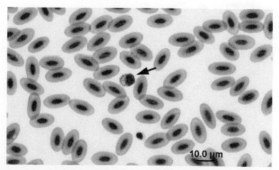

Fig. 6. Basophil (*arrow*) in the blood film of a hawk (*Buteo jamaicensis*) (Wright-Giemsa stain).

Lymphocyte

Lymphocytes are second only to the heterophil in frequency in most species except in Amazon parrots and some passerines (canaries). These species are often called "lymphocytic" because lymphocytes appear to be the predominate WBC and may account for up to 70% of circulating leukocytes.[3,7] Lymphocytes are typically round cells with a large nucleus-to-cytoplasmic ratio, but they may be somewhat irregular in shape due to molding around adjacent cells.[1] Lymphocytes have a round, centrally located, or slightly eccentric nuclei with densely clumped or reticulate nuclear chromatin and high nuclear-to-cytoplasmic (N/C) ratio (**Fig. 7**).[1,3] Their cytoplasm is clear or slightly basophilic and homogeneous, with no vacuolization.[2,3] Lymphocytes are usually characterized as small, medium, or large. Small or medium lymphocytes are the most common of the 3 in the peripheral blood. Small lymphocytes may be difficult to distinguish from avian thrombocytes, which have a clear, lightly blue or pale gray-colored cytoplasm, vacuolization, a larger more rounded darkly basophilic nucleus, and 2 small basophilic inclusions at the poles.[1–3] Reactive lymphocytes are medium to large in size with densely clumped chromatin, a deeply basophilic cytoplasm, a distinct pale Golgi zone, and cytoplasmic vacuoles.[1–3,6,7] Reactive lymphocytes may be present in small number in the peripheral blood smear and indicate antigenic stimulation often due to infectious diseases such as viral diseases (herpes virus or circovirus), chlamydophila infections, aspergillosis, tuberculosis, and salmonellosis.[2,6,7] Large lymphocytes with smooth disperse chromatin, nucleoli, abundant blue cytoplasm, and a prominent Golgi zone can be neoplastic and an indication of lymphoid leukemia or a leukemic phase of lymphoma.[3]

Lymphocytosis is not a common occurrence in birds, although an apparent increase may be seen in the previously mentioned "lymphocytic" species.[7] Lymphocytosis may result from antigenic stimulation of the immune system associated with infectious or inflammatory conditions or lymphocytic leukiemia.[3,15,18]

Lymphopenia may occur relative to a marked increase in heterophils.[6,7,15] More commonly, lymphopenia may result from excessive endogenous or exogenous corticosteroids, and viral infections and diseases that cause bursal damage or bone marrow suppression (pancytopenia).[1,3]

Monocyte

Monocytes are the largest of the mononuclear leukocytes, but are rarely seen in peripheral blood smears.[7] They are most often confused with large lymphocytes.

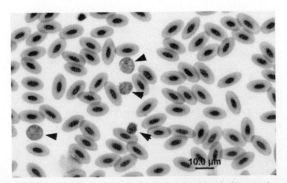

Fig. 7. Lymphocytes (*arrowheads*) in the blood film of a hawk (*Buteo jamaicensis*) (Wright-Giemsa stain).

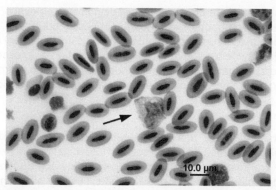

Fig. 8. Monocyte (*arrow*) in the blood film of a hawk (*Buteo jamaicensis*) (Wright-Giemsa stain).

Monocytes are round or amorphously shaped, with eccentric nuclei that are round, elongated, or indented, and the cytoplasm typically stains a blue-gray color with occasional vacuoles and fine eosinophilic granules (**Fig. 8**).[1–3,7] Monocytes are phagocytic, and once they enter into tissues they are transformed into macrophages.[3] Chlamydophila infections, and other chronic infectious diseases, such as tuberculosis, mycoses, and bacterial granulomatous diseases, are often but not always characterized by a monocytosis.[1,7,15] Monocytosis and basophilia have been described as the only hematological abnormalities seen in budgerigars with chlamydial infections. Because monocytes are not common in the peripheral blood, low or zero counts are not uncommon.[1,7]

Thrombocyte

Thrombocytes are small, oval or round cells, with dense nuclear chromatin, clear, faintly blue or pale gray cytoplasm, and one or more distinct granules at the poles (**Fig. 9**).[2,3,6,7] Thrombocytes are smaller than erythrocytes; however, they have a high N/C ratio and the nucleus is more rounded than that of erythrocytes. Avian thrombocytes arise from a stem cell, in contrast to mammalian platelets, which arise from megakaryocytes.[1,3,7] Thrombocyte counts are not commonly done, but instead, thrombocytes are reported as either adequate, increased, or decreased. The function of avian thrombocytes is not completely clear; however, they function in hemostasis

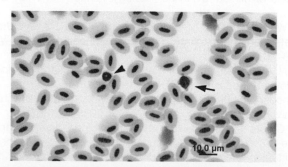

Fig. 9. Lymphocyte (*arrow*) and thrombocyte (*arrowhead*) in the blood film of a parrot (*Poicephalus senegalus*) (Wright-Giemsa stain).

and also are considered to be phagocytic, assisting in the removal of foreign material within the blood.[3,19] Thrombocytosis, although not well documented, may arise as an appropriated response to thrombocytopenia or chronic inflammatory disease in birds. Thrombocytopenia may occur due to increased destruction or excessive demand, as in septicemia or disseminated intravascular coagulation, bone marrow suppression (pancytopenia), and in some viral diseases (circovirus, reovirus, or polyomavirus).[1,7]

SUMMARY

Avian veterinarians often rely heavily on the results of various diagnostic tests, including hematology results. As such, cellular identification and evaluation of the cellular response are invaluable tools that help veterinarians understand the health or condition of their patient, as well as to monitor severity and clinical progression of disease and response to treatment. Therefore, it is important to thoroughly understand how to identify and evaluate changes in the avian erythron and leukon, as well as to interpret normal and abnormal results.

REFERENCES

1. Campbell TW, Ellis CK. Hematology of birds. In: Campbell TW, Ellis CK, editors. Avian and exotic animal hematology and cytology. 3rd edition. Ames (IA): Blackwell Publishing Professional; 2007. p. 3–50.
2. Doneley B. Interpreting diagnostic tests. In: Avian medicine and surgery in practice: companion and aviary birds. London: Manson Publishing Ltd; 2011. p. 69–91.
3. Mitchell EB, Johns J. Avian hematology and related disorders. Vet Clin North Am Exot Anim Pract 2008;11:501–22.
4. Herbert R, Nanney J, Spano JS, et al. Erythrocyte distribution in ducks. Am J Vet Res 1989;50:958–60.
5. Jones MP, Arheart KL, Cray C. Reference intervals, longitudinal analyses, and index of individuality of commonly measured laboratory variables in captive bald eagles (*Haliaeetus leucocephalus*). J Avian Med Surg 2014;28:118–26.
6. Fudge AM. Avian complete blood count. In: Fudge AM, editor. Laboratory medicine: avian and exotic pets. Philadelphia: WB Saunders Co; 2000. p. 9–18.
7. Fudge AM. Avian clinical pathology—hematology and chemistry. In: Altman RB, Clubb SL, Dorrestein GM, et al, editors. Avian medicine and surgery. Philadelphia: WB Saunders Co; 1997. p. 142–57.
8. Clark P, Boardman WSJ, Raidal SR. General hematological characteristics of birds. In: Atlas of clinical avian hematology. Ames (IA): Wiley-Blackwell; 2009. p. 33–53.
9. Campbell TW. Hematology of psittacines. In: Weiss DJ, Wardrop KJ, editors. Schalm's veterinary hematology. 6th edition. Hoboken (NJ): Wiley-Blackwell; 2010. p. 968–76.
10. Campbell TW. Avian hematology. In: Avian hematology and cytology. 2nd edition. Ames (IA): Iowa State University Press; 1995. p. 3–19.
11. Johns JL, Shooshtari MP, Christopher MM. Development of a technique for quantification of avian reticulocytes. Am J Vet Res 2008;69:1067–72.
12. Capitelli R, Crosta L. Overview of psittacine blood analysis and comparative retrospective study of clinical diagnosis, hematology and blood chemistry in selected psittacine species. Vet Clin North Am Exot Anim Pract 2013;16:71–120.
13. Johnston MS, Son TT, Rosenthal KL. Immune-mediated hemolytic anemia in an eclectus parrot. J Am Vet Med Assoc 2007;230:1028–31.

14. Campbell TW. Hematology. In: Ritchie BW, Harrison GJ, Harrison LR, editors. Avian medicine: principles and applications. Lake Worth (FL): Wingers Publishing; 1994. p. 176–98.
15. Fudge AM, Joseph V. Disorders of avian leukocytes. In: Fudge AM, editor. Laboratory medicine: avian and exotic pets. Philadelphia: WB Saunders Co; 2000. p. 19–25.
16. Scope A, Filip T, Gabler C, et al. The influence of stress from transport and handling on hematologic and clinical chemistry blood parameters of racing pigeons (*Columbia livia domestica*). Avian Dis 2002;46:1224–9.
17. Woerpel RW, Rosskopf WJ. Clinical experience with avian laboratory diagnostics. Vet Clin North Am Small Anim Pract 1984;14(2):249–80.
18. Schoemaker NJ, Dorrestein GM, Latimer KS, et al. Severe leukopenia and liver necrosis in young African grey parrots (*Psittacus erithacus erithacus*) infected with psittacine circovirus. Avian Dis 2000;44(2):470–8.
19. Grecchi R, Saliba AM, Mariano M. Morphological changes, surface receptors and phagocytic potential of fowl mono-nuclear phagocytes and thrombocytes in vivo and in vitro. J Pathol 1980;130:23–31.

Reptile Hematology

John M. Sykes IV, DVM, DACZM[a],*,
Eric Klaphake, DVM, DACZM, DABVP (Avian), DABVP (Reptile/Amphibian)[b]

KEYWORDS

- Reptile • Hematology • Leukogram • Phlebotomy • Snake • Chelonian • Lizard
- Crocodilian

KEY POINTS

- Sample collection and processing: Most reptile species have accessible sites for blood sample collection. The anticoagulant of choice is heparin, although slides made from fresh nonanticoagulated blood are best if possible. Syringes and needles can be coated with heparin before collection to prevent clotting in small patients. A Romanowsky-type stain is preferred for cytology (eg, Giemsa). Rapid stains can be used to produce acceptable hemogram results but may understain some cell types.
- Lymph contamination: In most reptiles, the lymphatic drainage system is closely paired with the venous system such that lymph contamination of blood samples is a common occurrence. Grossly contaminated samples should not be used for hematology. In addition, samples with low packed cell volume, no evidence of regeneration (polychromasia), and a high percentage of small lymphocytes are likely to be significantly lymph contaminated, and the hemogram results should be interpreted with caution.
- Variation: The normal hemogram of reptiles varies by many factors including species, age, gender, season, environmental parameters, geographic location, and sample collection method. Because of this variation, values should be compared with reference intervals most closely matching the species and situation for each individual reptile. As these values are often not available, interpretation of the hemogram may rely heavily on cell morphology and on changes over the progression of a disease rather than on absolute values at a single point in time.

INTRODUCTION

The basic principles of hematology used in mammalian medicine can be applied to reptiles. This article outlines techniques for sample collection, processing, and analysis that are unique to reptiles, and provides a review of factors influencing interpretation of the results.

[a] Zoological Health Program, Wildlife Conservation Society, Bronx Zoo, 2300 Southern Boulevard, Bronx, NY 10460, USA; [b] Cheyenne Mountain Zoo, 4250 Cheyenne Mountain Zoo Road, Colorado Springs, CO 80906, USA
* Corresponding author.
E-mail address: jsykes@wcs.org

Vet Clin Exot Anim 18 (2015) 63–82
http://dx.doi.org/10.1016/j.cvex.2014.09.011
1094-9194/15/$ – see front matter © 2015 Elsevier Inc. All rights reserved.

RESTRAINT AND BLOOD COLLECTION TECHNIQUES
General Comments

Before collecting a blood sample, the maximum safe volume that can be collected should be determined. Reptiles have a lower total blood volume than a similarly sized mammal, 5% to 8% of their body weight,[1,2] and 10% of this volume may be safely collected from healthy reptiles (eg, 0.5–0.8 mL in a 100-g animal). Smaller samples should be collected from compromised individuals.

Lithium heparin is generally the anticoagulant of choice in reptiles, as ethylenediaminetetraacetic acid (EDTA) has been reported to cause hemolysis, particularly in chelonians.[3,4] However, other studies of multiple reptilian species that suggest EDTA produces blood smears of comparable or better quality to those using heparin.[5–8] Ideally, hematology slides should be prepared from samples immediately after collection to avoid complications related to the anticoagulant. However, when drawing a sample from small individuals, it can be helpful to heparinize the needle and syringe before collection to prevent clot formation in the syringe. A study of slide preparation using blood obtained from green iguanas (Iguana iguana)[9] found that both the coverslip-slide method and bevel-edge slide techniques produced adequate quality smears, whereas the slide-slide method produced lower quality smears (higher numbers of ruptured cells). Slides are stained with a Romanowsky-type stain for morphologic analysis (eg, Giemsa, Wright, or Wright-Giemsa).[10,11] Rapid stains, such as Diff-Quik, may result in understaining or damage to some cell types, but can be used to produce adequate hemogram results.[11] For all venipuncture attempts, cleaning the skin with a dilute chlorhexidine solution before phlebotomy is prudent.

Snakes

There are 2 common venipuncture sites in snakes: the caudal tail vein (**Fig. 1**) and the heart (**Fig. 2**).[12,13] For either site, proper restraint of the snake's head is critical for handler safety. The caudal tail vein is accessed by holding the snake in dorsal recumbency and stabilizing the tail caudal to the cloaca. Holding the tail ventral to the body, such as over the end of a table, aids in successful collection. The needle is inserted on the midline between one-third and one-half the distance from the cloaca to the tip of the tail (usually 6–12 scutes caudal to the cloaca) at a 45° angle directed cranially. Avoid puncture of the hemipenes and scent glands that lie on either side of the midline. The needle is advanced with slight negative pressure. If vertebrae are encountered,

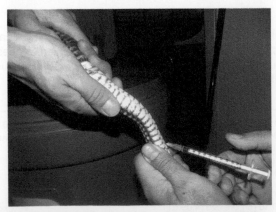

Fig. 1. Blood collection from the tail vein of a snake (Naja kaouthia).

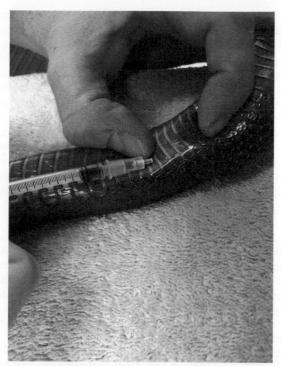

Fig. 2. Blood collection from the heart of a snake (unknown species).

the needle should be backed out and redirected. Restraint for this site is easy, but it can be difficult to collect a large volume from the tail, and risks include lymphatic contamination and trauma or infection to the hemipenes or scent glands. This site is useful for larger snakes and rattlesnakes, but is often more difficult to access in some colubrids and smaller boids.

For direct cardiac puncture, the snake is restrained in dorsal recumbency. The heart is usually located one-fourth to one-third the distance from the head to the tail.[12,14] It is found by visual inspection, palpation, or occasionally an ultrasound probe, particularly in larger snakes. Stabilize the heart with a finger cranial and the thumb caudal to the heart, taking care not to apply too much pressure, which may occlude blood flow in and out of the heart. The needle is inserted at a 45° angle into the ventricle of the heart. The syringe will fill slowly with each heart beat using only minimal negative pressure. Moderate digital pressure for up to 1 minute after the needle is withdrawn can decrease hematoma formation.[12] This technique can be performed safely in nonsedated snakes with adequate restraint provided the needle is minimally moved when in the body, although cardiac tamponade can occur if significant amounts of blood fill the pericardial space after puncture. If redirection is required, the needle should be withdrawn to the skin, redirected, and then advanced again.

Venipuncture of the palatine vein of snakes[15] is not recommended because of difficulties in restraint, minimal blood flow, and significant hematoma formation.

Lizards

Blood collection in lizards is usually from the tail vein with the lizard restrained in ventral or dorsal recumbency. Species that perform tail autotomy may need to be anesthetized (eg, with intramuscular ketamine)[16] before using this technique. One may also use the vagal technique (for calming lizards) by applying pressure over both eyes either digitally or by taping cotton balls over closed eyes. The tail vein can be accessed either ventrally or laterally. The ventral approach is performed as described for snakes. For the lateral approach, the needle is inserted at a 90° angle to the tail, just ventral to the lateral processes of the vertebrae, and directed medially. This site is identified by the longitudinal groove where the dorsal and ventral musculatures meet, although the groove can be difficult to locate on obese individuals.

The ventral abdominal vein lies within the coelomic cavity just dorsal to the ventral midline between the umbilicus and sternum. The lizard must be well restrained or anesthetized in dorsal recumbency, and the needle inserted along the ventral midline at a shallow angle and directed cranially. There is a risk of lacerating the vessel without the ability to apply pressure postprocedure, and puncture of other visceral structures is possible.[12,17]

Chelonians

Many venipuncture sites for chelonians have been described, including the heart; jugular, subcarapacial (**Fig. 3**), femoral, brachial (**Fig. 4**), and coccygeal veins (**Fig. 5**) and the occipital sinus.[12,18,19] The optimal site varies with the size and species, sedation level, medical condition, and experience of the phlebotomist. Samples collected from the jugular vein may be least likely to result in hemodilution because the vein can be visualized.[20] Regardless of site, pressure should be applied after collection for hemostasis.

The subcarapacial site is useful and easy to access in many species, particularly if access to the neck or limbs is difficult.[18,21] The head and neck can be either in extension or withdrawn into the shell. The needle is inserted on the midline where the skin of the neck meets the carapace. The exact angle of the needle to the body varies with the shape of the carapace, but is advanced along the ventral aspect of the carapace using mild negative pressure.[21] For larger animals, a spinal needle may be needed to reach the site. This site is the preferred alternative to toenail clipping for nonmedical personnel.[22]

Although the jugular vein may be preferred, its use is accompanied by difficult restraint. To access the site, the chelonian is positioned in ventral recumbency with the head held in a slightly more "head-down" position and with pressure applied to

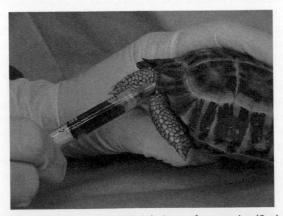

Fig. 3. Blood collection from the subcarapacial sinus of a tortoise (*Pyxis* sp). (*Courtesy of* Dr Bonnie L. Raphael, Bronx, NY.)

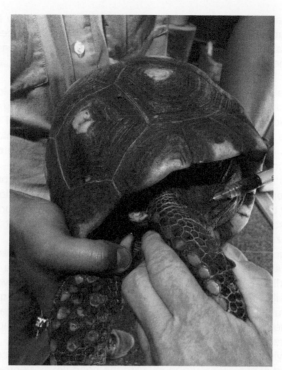

Fig. 4. Blood collection from the brachial plexus of a tortoise (*Chelonoidis carbonaria*). (*Courtesy of* Dr Bonnie L. Raphael, Bronx, NY.)

the back legs. The head is grasped using a ventral approach to avoid the normal defensive retraction response to dorsal threats. Grasping an extended foreleg prevents hinged tortoises from "boxing-up." Do not forcibly extract the head using instruments. Doing so can cause significant trauma to the beak. Once the head is restrained and extended, the vein is raised and visualized by applying pressure laterally at the thoracic inlet, either digitally or using a cotton-tipped applicator in smaller individuals.

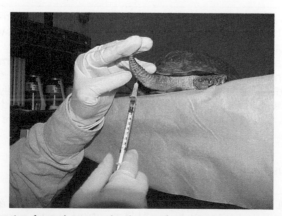

Fig. 5. Blood collection from the ventral tail vein of a turtle (unknown species). (*Courtesy of* Dr Bonnie L. Raphael, Bronx, NY.)

The presence and location of coccygeal veins in chelonians vary by species and may be dorsal, lateral, and/or ventral.[12] The dorsal vein can be accessed by flexing the tail ventrally and inserting the needle in a cranioventral direction as far cranially as possible on the dorsal midline. Lateral and ventral veins may be accessed with a technique similar to that already described for lizards.

The brachial vein (also called brachial plexus or ulnar plexus)[18] is located near the tendon of the triceps at the radiohumeral joint (elbow).[19] The foreleg is grasped and extended. The triceps tendon is palpated near the caudal aspect of the elbow joint, and the needle is inserted ventral to the tendon with the syringe held parallel to the forearm (see **Fig. 3**). Aldabra tortoises (*Geochelone gigantean*) have been trained for voluntary blood collection at this site.[23]

Cardiocentesis may be performed if other sites are not available, but in the clinical situation it is generally reserved for administration of euthanasia solution.[18,19] A needle is placed directly through the plastron on the midline near the junction of the pectoral and abdominal scutes.[12,19] Access via the thoracic inlet is difficult because of the inability to stabilize the heart and the required needle length.[19]

Two different approaches to the occipital sinus have been described.[19,24] In sternal recumbency, extend the head, aim the nose ventrally, then direct the needle caudally on the dorsal midline of the neck, just caudal to occiput.[19] Alternatively, position the chelonian vertically, extending and then flexing the head to make a 90° angle with the shell, and cranially direct the needle into the sinus at the dorsal midline of the neck.[24] With either method, a 25- or 23-gauge needle is used, and adequate manual or chemical restraint is critical.

The dorsal cervical sinuses (lateral occipital sinuses) are unique to sea turtles.[18] The turtle is restrained in sternal recumbency with the head flexed ventrally. The sinuses are dorsal and lateral to the cervical vertebrae. The needle is directed at up to a 90° angle into the sinus. These sinuses cannot be palpated and may be fairly deep (up to 3 cm).[13] Neck-restraining boxes and/or use of an ultrasound machine may help locate the proper site in larger sea turtles.

Sampling from cut toenails is not recommended. The sample size from this location will be small and contaminated with lymph, as the lymphatics of the area will be cut along with the blood vessels. This procedure is also considered to be painful, and may carry a greater risk of infection in comparison with collection from other sites.[13]

Crocodilians

The tail vein (**Fig. 6**) and the supravertebral sinus are the most commonly used sites in crocodilians. The tail vein is accessed as for lizards, either from a ventral or lateral approach. Collection from larger crocodilians can be facilitated by operant conditioning. The supravertebral sinus is accessed by restraining the animal in ventral recumbency with the head controlled. The needle (22- or 23-gauge) is placed on the ventral dorsal midline just caudal to the occiput and directed ventrally at a 90° angle. Negative pressure should be applied as the needle is advanced, and care should be taken, as spinal cord trauma (ie, pithing) can occur if needle is advanced too deeply.[12]

SAMPLE ANALYSIS
Erythrocytes

The packed cell volume (PCV), total erythrocyte count (RBC), and erythrocyte morphology should always be evaluated.[11,13] The PCV can be measured using hematocrit tubes as for mammals. The total RBC can be obtained using automated

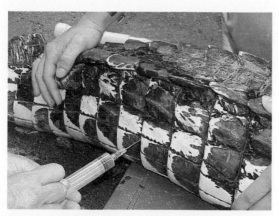

Fig. 6. Blood collection from the lateral approach to the tail vein on a crocodile (*Crocodylus rhombifer*). (*Courtesy of* Dr Bonnie L. Raphael, Bronx, NY.)

cell counters or manually.[25] Manual methods involve a hemocytometer and some type of staining/dilution system. The erythrocyte Unopette (Becton-Dickinson, Rutherford, NJ, USA) is one such system; an alternative system uses Natt and Herrick solution and a diluting pipette. Use of the Natt and Herrick solution allows determination of the RBC and total leukocyte count using the same sample in the hemocytometer.[10]

Mature reptilian erythrocytes are oval with an irregularly margined nucleus (**Figs. 7–15**).[10,11,26] New erythrocytes are created from the bone marrow, extramedullary sites such as the liver and spleen, or mature circulating cells dividing to form daughter cells.[10] Thus mitotic figures in circulating reptile erythrocytes may be normal. Compared with mature erythrocytes, immature cells appear smaller, rounder, have a basophilic cytoplasm, and have less dense chromatin in the nucleus (see **Fig. 7**).[11] Reticulocytes can be observed using a new methylene blue stain, and are 2.5% or less of the normal total RBC.[11] Hemoglobin, mean cell volume, and mean cell hemoglobin concentration are calculated as for mammals.

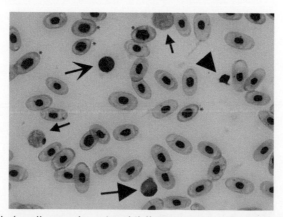

Fig. 7. Heterophils (*small arrows*), eosinophil (*large arrow*), azurophilic monocyte (*curved arrow*), lymphocyte (*arrowhead*), and immature erythrocytes (*asterisks*) in a bog turtle (*Glyptemys muhlenbergii*) (Diff-Quik stain, original magnification ×1000).

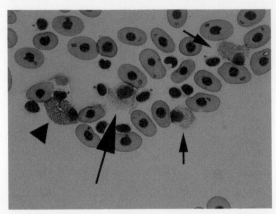

Fig. 8. Heterophils (*small arrows*), eosinophil (*arrowhead*), monocyte (*large arrow*), and thrombocytes (*asterisks*) in a tortoise (*Astrochelys radiata*) (Diff-Quik stain, original magnification ×1000).

Leukocytes

Complete leukocyte analysis includes a total leukocyte count (WBC), differential, and morphologic assessment.[11,13] Owing to the nucleated nature of reptile erythrocytes, automated methods of obtaining a WBC and differentials are not accurate. Manual methods for obtaining a WBC include estimated counts from blood smears, the semidirect method with phloxine B solution (eg, Unopette system), and the direct method (eg, using Natt and Herrick solution). Each method has advantages and disadvantages, and the accuracy of results depends on the cytologist's experience.

The estimated count method is performed by counting the total number of leukocytes in at least 10 fields of a stained blood smear using the high-dry (40× or 45×) objective. The average number of leukocytes per field is multiplied by 1500, resulting in the estimated leukocytes per microliter. This method is rapid and simple, but is prone to error if cells are clumped or not evenly distributed on the slide.[27]

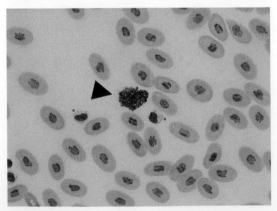

Fig. 9. Eosinophil (*arrowhead*) and thrombocytes (*asterisks*) of a pit viper (*Cryptelytrops macrops*) (Diff-Quik stain, original magnification ×1000).

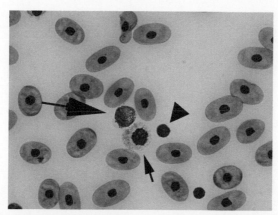

Fig. 10. Eosinophil (*large arrow*), basophil (*small arrow*), and a small lymphocyte (*arrowhead*) in a snapping turtle (*Chelydra serpentine*) (Diff-Quik stain, original magnification ×1000). Note that the basophil is understained using this staining technique.

The semidirect method is performed by staining acidophilic granulocytes with phloxine B solution. These stained granulocytes are counted in a hemocytometer, and a differential cell count is performed on a stained slide. The total WBC is then calculated using the number of heterophils and eosinophils counted in the hemocytometer and the percentage of such cells on the differential: Total WBC/μL = number of cells stained in hemocytometer chamber × 1.1 × 16 × 100/percentage of heterophils and eosinophils on differential.[25,28] This method requires an accurate differential for calculation of the WBC. If the heterophil count is low (due to true heteropenia or lysis of heterophils during creation of the blood smear), the total WBC can be artificially elevated.

The direct method is performed by staining all leukocytes with a solution such as Natt and Herrick, which are counted using a hemocytometer, and the total WBC is calculated. This method relies on distinguishing small lymphocytes from thrombocytes in the hemocytometer.[11,29] Inaccurately counting thrombocytes as lymphocytes will artificially elevate the result.

Heterophils (see **Figs. 7** and **8**) are the most common granulocyte in reptile blood and are analogous to the neutrophil.[10,13] Heterophils are round, may have

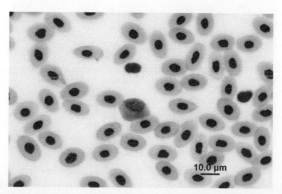

Fig. 11. An eosinophil with blue cytoplasmic granules in the blood film of a lizard (*Iguana iguana*) (Wright-Giemsa stain). (*Courtesy of* Dr Terry Campbell, Fort Collins, CO.)

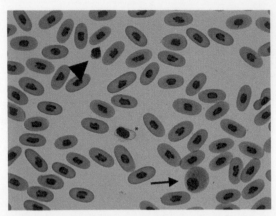

Fig. 12. Azurophil (*arrow*), lymphocyte (*arrowhead*), and thrombocyte (*asterisk*) in a python (*Morelia viridis*) (Diff-Quik stain, original magnification ×1000).

pseudopodia, and have clear cytoplasm.[10,13] The nucleus is round, eccentric, and may be bilobed.[13,29] The granules are eosinophilic, elongated, or spindle-shaped, and may be very numerous.[11,29] The morphology of heterophils may vary within an individual, particularly in the staining qualities of the granules. This variation has been hypothesized to be due to different stages of maturation of the heterophil, as this cell may mature while in circulation.[30–32] Toxic changes may be represented by the presence of a basophilic cytoplasm, abnormal granules, and vacuoles.[29,33] Degranulation may also be an indication of toxicity, although it may also be an artifact. A left shift may be indicated by the presence of myelocytes and metamyelocytes in circulation.[13] The presence of intracellular bacteria within leukocytes may indicate infection (see **Fig. 14**).

Eosinophils (see **Figs. 7–11**) are of similar size and shape to heterophils, and an eccentric nucleus is present. The distinguishing morphologic feature is that the eosinophilic granules of eosinophils are usually spherical, rather than the oval or elongated granules of heterophils.[10,11,29] Eosinophils of green iguanas (*I iguana*) are unusual because of their bluish-green spherical granules, the function of which is unknown

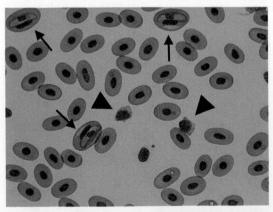

Fig. 13. Hemogregarine parasites within erythrocytes (*arrows*), lymphocytes (*arrowheads*), and a thrombocyte (*asterisk*) in a rattlesnake (*Crotalus horridus*) (Diff-Quik stain, original magnification ×1000).

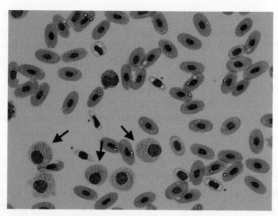

Fig. 14. Intracellular bacteria within azurophils (*arrows*), and thrombocytes (*asterisks*) in a python (*Python bivittatus*) (Diff-Quik stain, original magnification ×1000).

(see **Fig. 11**).[34] Eosinophils are not present in all species, particularly snakes[13]; they have been found in king cobras (*Ophiophagus hannah*),[32] but not in diamondback rattlesnakes (*Crotalus adamanteus*)[30] or yellow rat snakes (*Elaphae obsoleta quadrivitatta*).[8] Some investigators contend that eosinophils in snakes are actually variations of heterophils.[30] Variation of eosinophils within individuals, as described for heterophils, has been observed in green turtles (*Chelonia mydas*).[35]

Basophils (see **Fig. 10**) are small granulocytes with darkly basophilic granules that obscure the centrally located, nonlobed nucleus.[10,11] Care should be taken to distinguish between a normal basophil and a toxic heterophil where granules are basophilic and round.[29]

Lymphocytes (see **Figs. 7**, **10**, **12**, and **13**) of reptiles are morphologically similar to those of mammals. Lymphocytes lack granules, may be small or large, have a high nucleus to cytoplasm ratio, and have basophilic cytoplasm.[11,26] These cells may have phagocytosed particles or erythrocytes,[10,29] and typically contour to the shape of adjacent cells.[8,29] Reactive lymphocytes may indicate antigenic stimulation and are typically larger, with more basophilic cytoplasm that may contain discrete punctuate vacuoles.[13]

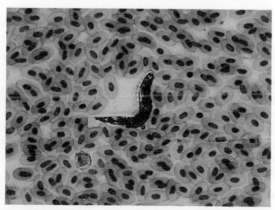

Fig. 15. Filarid nematode in a monitor lizard (*Varanus* sp) (Diff-Quik stain, original magnification ×1000).

Monocytes (see **Figs. 7** and **8**) are also similar to those of mammals. Monocytes are often the largest leukocyte (species dependent), with variably shaped contour and nucleus.[11,13] Monocytes of many nonsquamate reptiles contain azurophilc granules. These cells may be reported as "azurophils" or "azurophilic monocytes" but are a variation of the normal monocyte rather than a distinct cell type.[11,34] By contrast, azurophils of snakes (see **Figs. 12** and **14**) are a distinct cell type whose function is similar to that of the neutrophil.[30] The azurophils of snakes have finer granules and round nuclei in comparison with the azurophilic monocytes of other reptiles that have coarser granules and a lobulated nucleus.[36] Reactive monocytes may contain cytoplasmic vacuoles.[37]

Thrombocytes (see **Figs. 8**, **9**, **12**, **13**, and **14**) are small, oval basophilic cells with a central basophilic nucleus and pale-blue or colorless cytoplasm.[10,11] It is important to distinguish between small lymphocytes and thrombocytes when performing differential counts or using the direct method of obtaining the total WBC (see **Fig. 13**). Small lymphocytes are more round, with darker cytoplasm and more clumped chromatin in their nuclei in comparison with thrombocytes.[13,29]

FACTORS AFFECTING THE NORMAL HEMOGRAM

Species, slide staining and evaluation technique, health status, nutritional status, age, reproductive status, stress levels, gender, venipuncture site, season, hibernation status, captivity status, and environmental factors can affect the values and the presentation of blood cells. It is important to compare results from an individual with reference intervals that most closely match that individual. The following examples from recent articles highlight the range in variation within species, and demonstrate that these changes are not consistent across species or different situations.

Demographics

In a study of yellow-headed temple turtles (*Hieremys annandalii*), males were found to have higher WBC in comparison with females.[38] By contrast, a study of free-ranging cobras (*Naja naja*) found that females had higher WBC than did males.[39] The relative numbers of leukocytes may be different across genders, as demonstrated in yellow-marginated box turtles (*Cuora flavomarginata*) where males had higher eosinophil counts and females had higher monocyte counts.[40] Age may also play a role in altering parameters. For a population of loggerhead sea turtles (*Caretta caretta*), PCV and WBC were both lower in younger animals than in older juveniles. The differential counts were also different across ages, with younger animals having lower lymphocytes and higher granulocytes compared with older animals, and monocytes were lower in older animals.[41]

Biological Activity

In one study, nesting female leatherback turtles (*Dermochelys coriacea*) had lower eosinophil percentages than green (*C mydas*) and loggerhead turtles (*C caretta*). This finding was attributed to lower helminth parasite loads in leatherbacks resulting from their diet of jellyfish.[42] Another study comparing foraging, nesting, and stranded loggerhead sea turtles found significant differences between the groups for PCV and lymphocyte, monocyte, and total WBC counts.[43]

Season and Environmental Conditions

Environmental parameters affect the hemogram, but unfortunately changes are not always predictable. For example, PCV increases in desert tortoises (*Gopherus agassizii*) during dry periods,[44] similar to findings in yellow-marginated box turtles (*C flavomarginata*) whereby PCV was highest in summer months. These turtles also had lower monocyte counts in the summer.[40] By contrast, a study of Asian yellow pond turtles (*Ocadia sinensis*) found that all hematology parameters except monocytes varied with the season.[45] Differences can be found across a geographic range even for the same species and season. The numbers of heterophils, basophils, and azurophils varied across different locations for free-ranging giant garter snakes (*Thamnophis gigas*).[46] Captive reptiles may have values different from those of free-ranging individuals of the same species. For example, in Mediterranean pond turtles (*Mauremys leprosa*), the percentage of lymphocytes was 4.2% to 7.7% in free-ranging animals but 64.9% to 57.8% in captive animals, compared with 4.2% to 7.7% in free-ranging turtles.[47]

Restraint

Another factor to consider is immobilization or restraint of the reptile. Stress was induced in captive estuarine crocodiles (*Crocodylus porosus*) by 2 different handling methods: manual restraint (noosing with ropes) and immobilization by electrostunning. The investigators found that both groups showed a significant increase in PCV and hemoglobin concentration; however, the magnitude of change was significantly reduced and recovery was faster in stunned animals.[48] Another study found higher basophil counts in anesthetized free-ranging carpet pythons (*Morelia spilota imbricata*) when compared with those manually restrained.[49]

DISORDERS OF HEMATOLOGY

Much of the literature regarding the interpretation of reptilian hematologic results and their etiology is anecdotal and based on mammalian assumptions. Association of etiology with diagnostic results and correct treatment are often lacking in the peer-reviewed literature. What follows are personal anecdotal observations combined with reports from the literature when applicable.

Erythrocytic Disorders

Anemia

Because lymphatic vessels/sinuses usually run in tandem with veins, lymphodilution can occur with any sample. Even cardiocentesis can have contamination/dilution with pericardial fluid. Removal of some of the lymph in a particular venipuncture site before withdrawal of the needle may result in a "cleaner" sample on the next venipuncture attempt from the same site. Grossly contaminated samples are easily recognized and should be discarded. However, in other situations the degree of lymph contamination may be difficult to determine. In general, if the PCV is decreased (especially <15%), there is no evidence of regeneration (no polychromasia), and there are increased small lymphocytes in the sample, the degree of contamination is high and hematology results are likely invalid.

Because of this high frequency of hemodilution when collecting reptilian samples, the diagnosis of anemia may be difficult to make. If artifactual causes have been ruled out, true anemia may be due to blood loss, destruction, or decreased production. In many cases, a thorough history will suggest whether acute blood loss has occurred, such as from trauma. The presence of regeneration may be determined based on the degree of polychromasia, but reptile RBC are long-lived (up to 600–800 days)[50] and so the regenerative response is muted in comparison with mammals or birds. Anemia attributable to decreased production from chronic disease is the most common cause seen by the authors, as reptiles are often debilitated for an extended time before clinical signs are seen and veterinary care is sought. Causes for chronic anemia are many and may include infection, chronic exposure to improper environment and diet, chronic organ failure, toxin exposure, or neoplasia.

Polycythemia

Polycythemia has been suggested when the PCV exceeds 40%.[11] The most common cause is dehydration. One of the authors has encountered several cases of reptiles with PCV of this level and higher, many with concurrent elevations of total proteins or solids. Tentative diagnosis of dehydration has been made in these individuals, often subclinical, but polycythemia has also been noted in healthy reproductively active female iguanas (Klaphake, personal observation).

Inclusions

Erythrocyte inclusion bodies may be due to artifact from staining, viral particles, or the presence of hemoparasites (see **Fig. 13**). Iridovirus-related inclusion bodies have been observed incidentally and as causes of anemia in reptiles. In a fer-de-lance (*Bothrops moojeni*) evaluated for renal carcinoma, erythrocytes contained 2 types of inclusions, 1 viral and 1 crystalline. The snake was markedly anemic and exhibited a strong regenerative response. Ultrastructural analysis identified the virus to be an iridovirus consistent with snake erythrocyte virus, and the crystalline structures to be of a different nature to hemoglobin.[51] Inclusions of viral particles consistent with iridovirus have also been found in the erythrocytes and erythroblasts of free-ranging northern water snakes (*Nerodia sipedon sipedon*) from Canada[52] and free-ranging flap-necked chameleons (*Chamaeleo dilepis*) from Tanzania.[53]

The presence of hemoparasites has often been noted in nonclinical captive animals, leading to questions of their significance in captive reptiles.[54] Several free-ranging snakes in Florida inhabit the same environment with distinctive *Hepatozoon* species characteristic of each host species, none of which had apparent clinical signs.[55] There are, however, reports of disorder caused by hemoparasites. For example, blood cell composition (percent of immature erythrocytes) and blood hemoglobin were altered by infection with *Plasmodium* spp (severity varied depending on species of parasite) in eastern Caribbean island anoles (*Anolis sabanus*). Substantial data on 2 other lizard-malaria systems, *Sceloporus occidentalis* infected with *Plasmodium mexicanum* in northern California and *Agama agama* infected with *Plasmodium giganteum* and *Plasmodium agamae* in Sierra Leone, showed malaria was virulent in those 2 species as well.[56] In addition, hemogregarine parasites were thought to increase the monocyte count in a study of free-ranging lizards (*Ameiva ameiva*).[57] Fortunately, as many hemoparasites require an invertebrate as part of its life cycle, captive-raised reptiles, unless housed outdoors, seem to be at low risk for infection by these parasites.

Leukocytic Disorders

Infection is a challenging diagnosis to make in reptiles based on a single leukogram. Leukopenia, leukocytosis, and even a normal leukogram can all be present during infection. For example, in a study of siadenovirus in Sulawesi tortoises (*Indotestudo forsteni*), changes in affected animals included anemia, leukopenia or leukocytosis, heteropenia or heterophilia, lymphopenia or lymphocytosis, eosinophilia, and azurophilic monocytosis.[58] In another study of free-living spiny-tailed lizards (*Uromastyx* spp), one animal with a compound fracture of the humerus and associated abscess and osteolysis had an elevated RBC, leukocytosis, and heterophilia, whereas another individual with osteomyelitis of the stifle had a low RBC and leukopenia.[59] As with anemia, many illnesses in reptiles are due to chronic disease, whereby the WBC would be expected change over time and may regress back into a normal or leukopenic range through the weeks or months before presentation. This observation may explain the variation in leukocyte counts in the aforementioned examples.

Leukocytosis

As already mentioned, leukocytosis in reptiles is often associated anecdotally with infection. Elevated total WBC may reflect inflammation/immune response, infection, and/or stress. Following the WBC in an individual over time may be of more value than a single point sample. For example, in a study of cold-stunned Kemp's ridley turtle (*Lepidochelys kempii*), total WBC in convalescent animals were lower than those of cold-stunned animals, suggesting that as animals improved their WBC decreased.[60]

Often the more important parameters to interpret in the WBC are the differential and leukocyte morphology, rather than total WBC. For example, in a study of captive green turtles (*C mydas*) with or without ulcerative dermatitis, there was no difference seen in total WBC, but the heterophil/lymphocyte ratio was significantly increased in affected turtles. Along with a reduced delayed-type hypersensitivity reaction, it was postulated that the affected turtles were immunosuppressed.[61] Changes in the hemogram over time may also be important to monitor. In a study of the pathology associated with implanting radiotransmitters in eastern massasauga rattlesnakes (*Sistrurus catenatus catenatus*), all implanted animals had elevated heterophil and basophil counts 1 month after surgery. In one implanted group, this pattern had changed to higher lymphocyte counts many months later.[62] Reptilian monocytosis often is observed in immune responses to bacterial infections and parasitic infestations that result in tissue granuloma formation,[63] and eosinophilia may occasionally be caused by parasite infestation.[64]

Documented cases of leukocytosis have also been reported to be due to neoplastic leukemias. Hematopoietic malignancies are most commonly reported in lizards[65] and snakes,[66] occurring sporadically in other reptiles. These neoplasias may present as multiple discrete masses, such as with lymphosarcoma, as circulating neoplasms (leukemia), or as a combination of both forms.[63,67–69] Typically they occur as sporadic cases, but outbreaks or clusters of lymphoid neoplasms have been reported.[70]

Leukopenia

Leukopenia caused by toxicosis associated with fenbendazole was noted in a 125-day study of Hermann's tortoises (*Testudo hermanni*). Serial blood samples found that although the tortoises remained healthy, an extended heteropenia occurred. It was suggested that the risk of mortality of an individual from nematode infection should be assessed relative to the potential for metabolic alteration and secondary septicemia following damage to hematopoietic and gastrointestinal systems by fenbendazole.[71]

Inclusions/hemoparasites

As with erythrocytic inclusions, the differentials of artifact, virus, and hemoparasite should be considered. A free-ranging adult female eastern box turtle (*Terrapene carolina*) had intracytoplasmic inclusions consistent with iridovirus within heterophils and large mononuclear leukocytes on routine blood smear examination.[72] In a report of blood films examined from 170 specimens of 15 *Chamaeleo* spp in Tanzania, 3 *C dilepis* had an intracytoplasmic inclusion within monocytes. One of the lizards was maintained in captivity and, at 46 days, a second type of inclusion was occasionally seen within monocytes. Transmission electron microscopic examination of monocytes revealed the presence of a chlamydia-like organism and pox-like virus.[73]

ACKNOWLEDGMENTS

The authors thank Karen Ingerman, LVT, for her help with image acquisition and assistance with this article. This article was adapted from a previous version written by the authors: Reptile hematology. In: Hematology and related disorders. Vet Clin Exp Anim Pract 2008; 11.

REFERENCES

1. Lillywhite HB, Smits AW. Lability of blood volume in snakes and its relation to activity and temperature. J Exp Biol 1984;110:267–74.
2. Smits AW, Kozubowski MM. Partitioning of body fluids and cardiovascular responses to circulatory hypovolemia in the turtle Pseudemys scripta elegans. J Exp Biol 1985;116:237–50.
3. Jacobson ER. Blood collection techniques in reptiles. In: Fowler ME, editor. Zoo and wild animal medicine, current therapy 3. Philadelphia: WB Saunders Co; 1993. p. 144–52.
4. Muro J, Cuenca R, Pastor J, et al. Effects of lithium heparin and tripotassium EDTA on hematologic values of Hermann's tortoises (Testudo hermanni). J Zoo Wildl Med 1998;29(1):40–4.
5. Harr KE, Raskin RE, Heard DJ. Temporal effects of 3 commonly used anticoagulants on hematologic and biochemical variables in blood samples from macaws and Burmese pythons. Vet Clin Pathol 2005;34(4):383–8.
6. Hanley CS, Hernandez-Divers SJ, Bush S, et al. Comparison of the effect of dipotassium ethylenediaminetetraacetic acid and lithium heparin on hematologic values in the green iguana (Iguana iguana). J Zoo Wildl Med 2004;35(3):328–32.
7. Martinez-Jimenez D, Hernandez-Divers SJ, Floyd TM, et al. Comparison of the effects of dipotassium ethylenediaminetetraacetic acid and lithium heparin on hematologic values in yellow-blotched map turtles, Braptemys flavimaculata. J Herp Med Surg 2007;17(2):36–41.
8. Dotson TK, Ramsay ER, Bounous DI. A color atlas of blood cells of the yellow rat snake. Compend Contin Educ Pract Vet 1995;17:1013–6.
9. Perpinan D, Hernandez-Divers SM, McBride M, et al. Comparison of three different techniques to produce blood smears from green iguanas, Iguana iguana. J Herp Med Surg 2006;16(3):99–101.
10. Frye FL. Hematology as applies to clinical reptile medicine. In: Biomedical and surgical aspects of captive reptile husbandry. 2nd edition. Malabar (FL): Krieger Publishing Co; 1991. p. 209–79.
11. Campbell TW. Clinical pathology of reptiles. In: Mader DR, editor. Reptile medicine and surgery. 2nd edition. St Louis (MO): Saunders; 2006. p. 453–70.
12. Hernandez-Divers SJ. Diagnostic techniques. In: Mader DR, editor. Reptile medicine and surgery. 2nd edition. St Louis (MO): Saunders; 2006. p. 490–532.
13. Strik NI, Alleman AR, Harr KE. Circulating inflammatory cells. In: Jacobson ER, editor. Infectious diseases and pathology of reptiles color atlas and text. Boca Raton (FL): CRC Press; 2007. p. 167–218.
14. Jacobson ER. Overview of reptile biology, anatomy, and histology. In: Jacobson ER, editor. Infectious diseases and pathology of reptiles color atlas and text. Boca Raton (FL): CRC Press; 2007. p. 1–130.

15. Olson GA, Hessler JR, Faith RE. Techniques for blood collection and intravascular infusions of reptiles. Lab Anim Sci 1975;25:783–6.
16. Schumacher J, Yelen T. Anesthesia and analgesia. In: Mader DR, editor. Reptile medicine and surgery. 2nd edition. St Louis (MO): Saunders; 2006. p. 442–52.
17. Redrobe S, MacDonald J. Sample collection and clinical pathology of reptiles. Vet Clin North Am Exot Anim Pract 1999;2(3):709–30.
18. Barrows MS, McAurthur S, Wilkinson R. Diagnostics. In: McArthur S, Wilkinson R, Meyer J, editors. Medicine and surgery of tortoises and turtles. Oxford (United Kingdom): Blackwell Publishing Ltd; 2004. p. 109–40.
19. Lloyd M, Morris P. Chelonian venipuncture techniques. Bull Assoc Reptilian Amphibian Vet 1999;9(1):26–8.
20. Gottdenker NL, Jacobson ER. Effect of venipuncture sites on hematologic and clinical biochemical values in desert tortoises (*Gopherus agassizzi*). Am J Vet Res 1995;56:19–21.
21. Hernandez-Divers SM, Hernandaz-Divers SJ, Wyneken J. Angiographic, anatomic and clinical technique descriptions of a subcarapacial venipuncture site for chelonians. J Herp Med Surg 2002;21(2):32–7.
22. Johnson JD. Nail trimming for blood collection from desert tortoises, *Gopherus agassizii*: panel summary. J Herp Med Surg 2006;16(2):61–2.
23. Weiss W, Willson S. The use of classical and operant conditioning in training Aldabra tortoises (*Geochelone gigantean*) for venipuncture and other husbandry issues. J Appl Anim Welf Sci 2003;6(1):33–8.
24. Martinez-Silvestre A, Perpinan D, Marco I, et al. Venipuncture technique of the occipital venous sinus in freshwater aquatic turtles. J Herp Med Surg 2002; 12(4):31–2.
25. Pierson FW. Laboratory techniques for avian hematology. In: Feldman BF, Zinkl JG, Jain NC, editors. Schalm's veterinary hematology. 5th edition. Philadelphia: Lippincott Williams and Wilkins; 2000. p. 1145–7.
26. Saint Girons MC. Morphology of the circulating blood cell. In: Gans C, Parsons TC, editors. Biology of the reptilia, vol. 3. New York: Academic Press; 1970. p. 73–91.
27. Latimer KS, Bienzle D. Determination and interpretation of the avian leukogram. In: Feldman BF, Zinkl JG, Jain NC, editors. Schalm's veterinary hematology. 5th edition. Philadelphia: Lippincott Williams and Wilkins; 2000. p. 417–32.
28. Campbell TW. Avian hematology. In: Avian hematology and cytology. Ames (IA): Iowa State University Press; 1988. p. 3–17.
29. Wilkinson R. Clinical pathology. In: McArthur S, Wilkinson R, Meyer J, editors. Medicine and surgery of tortoises and turtles. Oxford: Blackwell Publishing Ltd; 2004. p. 141–86.
30. Alleman AR, Jacobson ER, Raskin RE. Morphological, cytochemical staining, and ultrastructural characteristics of blood cells from eastern diamondback rattlesnakes (*Crotalus adamaneus*). Am J Vet Res 1999;60:507–14.
31. Bounous DI, Dotson TK, Brooks RL, et al. Cytochemical staining and ultrastructural characteristics of peripheral blood leucocytes from the yellow rat snake (*Elaphe obsolete quadrivitatta*). Comp Haematol Int 1996;6:86–91.
32. Salakiji C, Salakij J, Apibal S, et al. Hematology, morphology, cytochemical staining, and ultrastructural characteristics of blood cells in king cobras (*Ophiophagus hannah*). Vet Clin Pathol 2002;31(3):116–26.
33. LeBlanc CJ, Heatley JJ, Mack EB. A review of the morphology of lizard leukocytes with a discussion of the clinical differentiation of bearded dragon, *Pogona vitticeps*, leukocytes. J Herp Med Surg 2000;19(2):27–30.

34. Harr KE, Alleman AR, Dennis PM, et al. Morphologic and cytochemical character-
    istics of blood cells and hematologic and plasma biochemical reference ranges
    in green iguanas. J Am Vet Med Assoc 2001;218(6):915–21.
35. Work TM, Raskin RE, Balazs GH, et al. Morphological and cytochemical charac-
    teristics of blood cells from Hawaiian green turtles. Am J Vet Res 1998;59:1252–7.
36. Alleman AR, Jacobson ER, Raskin RE. Morphologic and cytochemical character-
    istics of blood cells from the desert tortoise (Gopherus agassizii). Am J Vet Res
    1992;53:1645–51.
37. Stacy NI, Alleman AR, Sayler KA. Diagnostic hematology of reptiles. Clin Lab
    Med 2011;31:87–108.
38. Chansue N, Sailasuta A, Tangtrongpiros J, et al. Hematology and clinical chem-
    istry of adult yellow-headed temple turtles (Hieremys annandalii) in Thailand. Vet
    Clin Pathol 2011;40:174–84.
39. Parida SP, Dutta SK, Pal A. Hematology and plasma biochemistry of wild-caught
    Indian cobra Naja naja (Linnaeus, 1758). J Venom Anim Toxins Incl Trop Dis 2014;
    20:14.
40. Yang PY, Yu PH, Wu SH, et al. Seasonal hematology and plasma biochemistry refer-
    ence range values of the yellow-marginated box turtle (Cuora flavomarginata).
    J Zoo Wildl Med 2014;45:278–86.
41. Rousselet E, Stacy NI, LaVictoire K, et al. Hematology and plasma biochemistry
    analytes in five age groups of immature, captive-reared loggerhead sea turtles
    (Caretta caretta). J Zoo Wildl Med 2013;44:859–74.
42. Deem SL, Dierenfeld ES, Sounguet GP, et al. Blood values in free-ranging nesting
    leatherback sea turtles (Dermochelys coriacea) on the coast of the Republic of
    Gabon. J Zoo Wildl Med 2006;37(4):464–71.
43. Deem SL, Norton TM, Mitchell M, et al. Comparison of blood values in foraging,
    nesting, and stranded loggerhead turtles (Caretta caretta) along the coast of
    Georgia, USA. J Wildl Dis 2009;45:41–56.
44. Dickinson VM, Jarchow JL, Trueblood MH. Hematology and plasma biochemistry
    reference range values for free-ranging desert tortoises in Arizona. J Wildl Dis
    2002;38:143–53.
45. Chung CS, Cheng CH, Chin SC, et al. Morphologic and cytochemical charac-
    teristics of Asian yellow pond turtle (Ocadia sinensis) blood cells and their
    hematologic and plasma biochemical reference values. J Zoo Wildl Med
    2009;40:76–85.
46. Wack RF, Hansen E, Small M, et al. Hematology and plasma biochemistry
    values for the giant garter snake (Thamnophis gigas) and valley garter snake
    (Thamnophis sirtalis fitchi) in the Central Valley of California. J Wildl Dis 2012;
    48:307–13.
47. Hidalgo-Vila J, Diaz-Paniagua C, Perez-Santigosa N, et al. Hematologic and
    biochemical reference intervals of free-living Mediterranean pond turtles
    (Mauremys leprosa). J Wildl Dis 2007;43(4):798–801.
48. Franklin CE, Davis BM, Peucker SK, et al. Comparison of stress induced by
    manual restraint and immobilisation in the estuarine crocodile, Crocodylus
    porosus. J Exp Zool A Comp Exp Biol 2003;298(2):86–92.
49. Bryant GL, Fleming PA, Twomey L, et al. Factors affecting hematology and
    plasma biochemistry in the southwest carpet python (Morelia spilota imbricata).
    J Wildl Dis 2012;48:282–94.
50. Frye FL. Hematology as applied to clinical reptile medicine. In: Frye FL, editor.
    Biomedical and surgical aspects of captive reptile husbandry, vol. 1, 2nd edition.
    Melbourne (Australia): Krieger Publishing Cp; 1991. p. 209–77.

51. Johnsrude JD, Raskin RE, Hoge AY, et al. Intraerythrocytic inclusions associated with iridoviral infection in a fer de lance (*Bothrops moojeni*) snake. Vet Pathol 1997;34(3):235–8.
52. Smith TG, Desser SS, Hong H. Morphology, ultrastructure and taxonomic status of *Toddia* sp. in northern water snakes (*Nerodia sipedon sipedon*) from Ontario, Canada. J Wildl Dis 1994;30(2):169–75.
53. Telford SR, Jacobson ER. Lizard erythrocytic virus in East-African chameleons. J Wildl Dis 1993;29(1):57–63.
54. Campbell TW. Hemoparasites. In: Mader DR, editor. Reptile medicine and surgery. 2nd edition. St Louis (MO): Elsevier; 2006. p. 801–5.
55. Telford SR, Wozniak EJ, Butler JF. Haemogregarine specificity in two communities of Florida snakes, with descriptions of six new species of Hepatozoon (Apicomplexa: Hepatozoidae) and a possible species of *Haemogregarina* (Apicomplexa: Haemogregarinidae). J Parasitol 2001;87(4):890–905.
56. Schall JJ, Staats CM. Virulence of lizard malaria: three species of plasmodium infecting *Anolis sabanus*, the endemic anole of Saba, Netherlands Antilles. Copeia 2002;(1):39–43.
57. Bonadiman SF, Miranda FJ, Ribeiro ML, et al. Hematological parameters of *Ameiva ameiva* (Reptilia: Teiidae) naturally infected with hemogregarine: confirmation of monocytosis. Vet Parasitol 2010;171:146–50.
58. Rivera S, Wellehan JF, McManamon R, et al. Systemic adenovirus infection in Sulawesi tortoises (*Indotestudo forsteni*) caused by a novel siadenovirus. J Vet Diagn Invest 2009;21:415–26.
59. Naldo JL, Libanan NL, Samour JH. Health assessment of a spiny-tailed lizard (*Uromastyx* spp.) population in Abu Dhabi, United Arab Emirates. J Zoo Wildl Med 2009;40:445–52.
60. Innis CJ, Ravich JB, Tlusty MF, et al. Hematologic and plasma biochemical findings in cold-stunned Kemp's ridley turtles: 176 cases (2001-2005). J Am Vet Med Assoc 2009;235:426–32.
61. Muñoz FA, Estrada-Parra S, Romero-Rojas A, et al. Immunological evaluation of captive green sea turtle (*Chelonia mydas*) with ulcerative dermatitis. J Zoo Wildl Med 2013;44:837–44.
62. Lentini AM, Crawshaw GJ, Licht LE, et al. Pathologic and hematologic responses to surgically implanted transmitters in eastern massasauga rattlesnakes (*Sistrurus catenatus catenatus*). J Wildl Dis 2011;47:107–25.
63. Gregory CR, Latimer KS, Fontenot DK, et al. Chronic monocytic leukemia in an Inland Bearded Dragon, *Pogona vitticeps*. J Herp Med Surg 2004;14(2):12–6.
64. Hidalgo-Vila J, Martínez-Silvestre A, Ribas A, et al. Pancreatitis associated with the helminth *Serpinema microcephalus* (Nematoda: Camallanidae) in exotic red-eared slider turtles (*Trachemys scripta elegans*). J Wildl Dis 2011;47: 201–5.
65. Hernandez-Divers SM, Orcutt CJ, Stahl SJ, et al. Lymphoma in lizards—three case reports. J Herp Med Surg 2003;13(1):14–21.
66. Garner MM, Hernandez-Divers SM, Raymond JT. Reptile neplasia: a retrospective study of case submissions to a specialty diagnostic service. Vet Clin North Am Exot Anim Pract 2004;7(3):653–71.
67. Tocidlowski ME, McNamara PL, Wojcieszyn JW. Myelogenous leukemia in a bearded dragon (*Acanthodraco vitticeps*). J Zoo Wildl Med 2001;32(1):90–5.
68. Schultze AE, Mason GL, Clyde VL. Lymphosarcoma with leukemic blood profile in a Savannah monitor lizard (*Varanus exanthematicus*). J Zoo Wildl Med 1999; 30(1):158–64.

69. Schilliger L, Selleri P, Frye FL. Lymphoblastic lymphoma and leukemic blood profile in a red-tail boa (*Boa constrictor constrictor*) with concurrent inclusion body disease. J Vet Diagn Invest 2011;23:159–62.
70. Gyimesi ZS, Garner MM, Burns RB, et al. High incidence of lymphoid neoplasia in a colony of Egyptian spiny-tailed lizards (*Uromastyx aegyptius*). J Zoo Wildl Med 2005;36(1):103–10.
71. Neiffer DL, Lydick D, Burks K, et al. Hematologic and plasma biochemical changes associated with fenbendazole administration in Hermann's tortoises (*Testudo hermanni*). J Zoo Wildl Med 2005;36(4):661–72.
72. Allender MC, Fry MM, Irizarry AR, et al. Intracytoplasmic inclusions in circulating leukocytes from an eastern box turtle (*Terrapene carolina carolina*) with iridoviral infection. J Wildl Dis 2006;42(3):677–84.
73. Jacobson ER, Telford SR. Chlamydial and poxvirus infections of circulating monocytes of a flap-necked chameleon (*Chamaeleo dilepis*). J Wildl Dis 1990; 26:572–7.

Fish Hematology and Associated Disorders

Krystan R. Grant, DVM

KEYWORDS

- Fish • Teleost • Elasmobranch • Hematology • Erythrocytes • Leukocytes
- Thrombocytes • Blood cells

KEY POINTS

- This article reviews blood-collecting techniques including restraint, venipuncture sites, and sample handing.
- The section on hematologic evaluation includes the steps necessary to perform manual counts for total red and white blood cells, and cell descriptions for identification.
- Tables are included summarizing the reported etiology of changes in cell counts, packed cell volume, and red blood cell indices.

INTRODUCTION

There are scientific descriptions of approximately 27,300 different species of fish, which exceeds that of all other vertebrates combined.[1,2] With this many different types of known fish, the intrigue of their diversity is understandable. Ownership of captive pet fish shows an upward trend with approximately 148 million fish, or more than 41% of owned pets in the United States, in more than 69 million households.[3] In addition to pet fish, captivity also encompasses those in public aquaria, other educational facilities, and aquaculture. With the growing number and value of freshwater and marine fishes in captivity, the demand for their medical care increases. Fish handling, diagnostics, medicine, and surgery are often more challenging than in terrestrial and arboreal animals simply because of their aquatic nature.

One diagnostic tool that may assist the veterinary staff with detecting disease or identifying change is hematologic evaluation. As with other animals, normal variation from intrinsic or extrinsic factors or diseases affecting blood cells and counts may be evaluated by clinical hematology. Obtaining even a small blood sample may reveal information helpful in guiding treatment options.

The author has nothing to disclose.
Colorado State University, Department of Clinical Sciences, 300 West Drake Road, Fort Collins, CO 80523, USA
E-mail address: Krystan.grant@colostate.edu

Vet Clin Exot Anim 18 (2015) 83–103
http://dx.doi.org/10.1016/j.cvex.2014.09.007
1094-9194/15/$ – see front matter © 2015 Elsevier Inc. All rights reserved.

The volume of information pertaining to reference intervals and interpretation of blood test results is relatively limited, which is expected given the number of different fish. Other challenges involved with hematologic evaluation in fish include the differences between publications regarding the nomenclature and function of blood cells. Research is ongoing, and the purpose of this article is to summarize the value, technique, and general interpretation of fish hematology.

BLOOD COLLECTION
Restraint Techniques

Blood collection from fish may be accomplished with either physical or chemical restraint. Physical restraint is the method used if the patient is cooperative or severely debilitated, and when the clinician is comfortable doing so without causing a great amount of stress to the animal. The integument of fish provides many functions, and should be approached and handled with caution for protection of the fish and the handler. Appropriate gloves should be worn to protect the handler from zoonotic disease and from physical and chemical defense mechanisms of the fish, and to protect the mucous layer of the fish.[4] Most small fish can be approached by using one hand to grasp near the base of the tail while supporting the body with the other hand.[5,6] The use of ancillary equipment, such as nets or stretchers, may be required depending on the size of the animal (**Fig. 1**). Some elasmobranchs may enter a hypnotic state referred to as tonic immobility when placed in dorsal recumbency (**Fig. 2**).[7–10] Tonic immobility has been noted in several species, and offers a short duration of decreased activity allowing for minor procedures such as physical or ultrasonographic examination, venipuncture, or administration of medications.

When physical restraint cannot be accomplished and the animal can withstand anesthesia, chemical assistance typically is used. There are many agents used for fish anesthesia but one of the most commonly used Food and Drug Administration–approved agents is tricaine methanesulfonate (Tricaine-S, previously Finquel). Tricaine methanesulfonate is also commonly referred to as tricaine, TMS, MS-222, or triple-2. Tricaine requires buffering with 2 parts sodium bicarbonate and is used to create induction and anesthetic baths. Many factors, such as physical characteristics of the fish, environmental conditions, and the procedure, will contribute to the optimum dose and therefore should be considered before use. Suggested initial doses

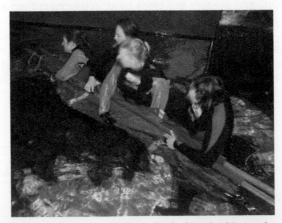

Fig. 1. Four aquarists restraining a sandbar shark (*Carcharhinus plumbeus*) in the red stretcher in preparation for examination.

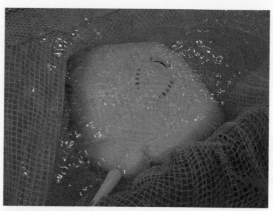

Fig. 2. Tonic immobility of a southern stingray (*Dasyatis americana*).

have been published (ranging from 50 to 400 mg/L), with a typical induction range for most fish at 50 to 150 mg/L, but it is recommended to begin conservatively.[10–15] A summary of the stages of anesthetic depths is provided in **Table 1**. Once the procedure is completed or nearly completed, the fish is gently ram-ventilated in appropriate untreated recovery water. Induction, anesthetic, and recovery baths should all be properly aerated.

Venipuncture Sites

A blood sample is often collected from the caudal vein by approaching it via the lateral or ventral tail. The lateral approach in teleosts (bony fish) begins with the fish in lateral recumbency and identification of the lateral line. An appropriately sized needle and syringe should be used. The needle is inserted into the skin between the scales, if applicable, just ventral to the lateral line. As the needle penetrates through the skin, mild negative pressure can be applied to the syringe as the needle is advanced deeper into the tissue until blood enters the syringe (**Fig. 3**). If bone is detected with the needle, the needle should be repositioned ventrally (below the spine). The ventral approach begins with the fish in dorsal recumbency. The needle is inserted on midline

Table 1			
Summary of stages of anesthetic depth when using MS-222 in fish			
Stage	**Response**	**Reaction to External Stimuli**	**Opercular Rate**
1	Light sedation	Slight loss	Slight decrease
2	Deep sedation	Total loss (except with strong pressure)	Slight decrease
3	Partial loss of equilibrium and muscle tone, hyperactive behavior	Total loss (except with strong pressure)	Increase
4	Total loss of equilibrium and muscle tone	Loss of spinal reflexes	Slow and regular
5	Loss of reflex activity	Total loss	Slow and irregular
6	None	None	Asphyxia, ceased

Data from Carter KM, Woodley CM, Brown RS. A review of tricaine methanesulfonate for anesthesia of fish. Rev Fish Biol Fisheries 2011;21(1):51–9.

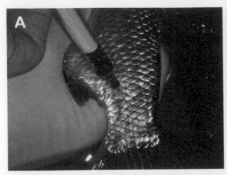
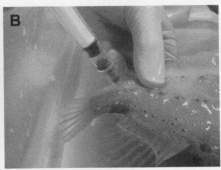

Fig. 3. (*A*) The tinfoil barb (*Barbonymus schwanenfeldii*) is in right lateral recumbency for collection of a blood sample from the caudal vein using the lateral approach. (*B*) The lumpfish (*Cyclopterus lumpus*) is in right lateral recumbency for collection of a blood sample from the caudal vein using the lateral approach.

of the ventral tail. Slight aspiration of the plunger is applied once the needle has penetrated the skin, and advanced deeper into the tissue until blood enters the syringe. Again, if bone is detected then the needle should be slightly retracted or repositioned left or right, depending on the position of the bone with respect to the needle.

Elasmobranch (cartilaginous fish) blood samples may also be collected from the caudal vein, and in larger sharks the dorsal venous sinus may be used. A ventral approach is often used with the animal in dorsal recumbency, the needle being inserted into the ventral midline of the tail. Once the needle has penetrated the skin, negative pressure is applied to the plunger. The needle is carefully advanced deeper into the tissue and possibly through a thin layer of cartilage to reach the vein (**Fig. 4**). Blood collection in larger sharks can be done at the dorsal venous sinus near the dorsal fin. With the shark in ventral recumbency, the caudal flap of the dorsal fin is lifted to expose the denticle-free skin. The needle is inserted in the center of the flesh pocket with negative pressure applied to the syringe. The needle may need to be repositioned or advanced to find the sinus (**Fig. 5**).

Cardiocentesis is another option for obtaining a blood sample, although this method may put the fish at a greater risk of injury or death.[16,17]

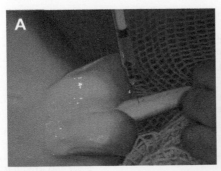
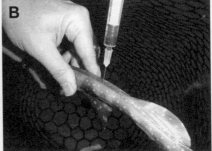

Fig. 4. (*A*) The southern stingray (*Dasyatis americana*) is in dorsal recumbency for collection of a blood sample from the caudal vein using the ventral approach. (*B*) The white-spotted bamboo shark (*Chiloscyllium plagiosum*) is in dorsal recumbency for collection of a blood sample from the caudal vein using the ventral approach.

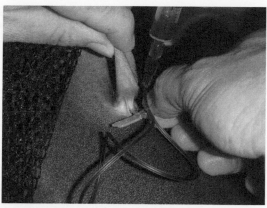

Fig. 5. The blacktip reef shark (*Carcharhinus melanopterus*) is in ventral recumbency for collection of a blood sample from the dorsal venous sinus.

Sample Handling

The amount of blood that can be safely obtained from a healthy fish has been reported at 30% to 50% of total blood volume.[18] Typically sample collection is approximately 1% of the body weight.[17,18] Once blood is retrieved it should be placed in a micro-tainer containing an anticoagulant, such as lithium heparin or ethylenediaminetetra-acetic acid (EDTA). For hematologic evaluation the preferred anticoagulant is species specific, although heparin seems to be most commonly used.[19,20] For elasmobranch blood, although heparin can be used, a combination of heparin and EDTA or use of another modified anticoagulant solution is ideal to match the osmolarity of the blood.[21] Preferably fresh blood smears should be made at the time of blood collection, although they may also be made from the collected sample in anticoagulant.

HEMATOLOGIC EVALUATION
Erythrocyte Structure and Function

Most fish have nucleated erythrocytes, the exceptions being the silvery lightfish (*Maurolicus muelleri*) and other members of the Gonostomidae family (*Valenciennellus tripunctatus* and *Vinciguerria* sp), which have anucleated erythrocytes.[2,22,23] The structure of erythrocytes in fish is generally oval to elliptical with a centrally positioned, basophilic nucleus and pale, slightly eosinophilic cytoplasm.[2,24,25] The number and size of erythrocytes vary among species, but elasmobranch red blood cells (RBCs) are generally larger and more rounded in comparison with bony fish.[2,25,26] It has been reported that erythrocyte size is proportional to its genome size (or nucleus size determined by the amount of deoxyribonucleic acid)[27] and inversely related to the standard metabolic rate.[28] The primary function of RBCs is oxygen transport, the extent of which depends on the amount of hemoglobin concentration within the cell and the gas-exchange mechanism.[22]

Approximately 1% of the peripheral RBC population may be immature erythrocytes, likely derived from circulatory erythropoiesis.[16] Immature erythrocytes will contribute to polychromasia and anisocytosis because of their smaller, round shape and dark-staining nucleus and cytoplasm in comparison with their mature counterparts. The nucleus to cytoplasm ratio is much greater in young RBCs and decreases as the cells mature, allowing the hemoglobin content to increase. Because the presence of immature erythrocytes in peripheral blood may be normal, noting it in cases of anemic fish does not necessarily translate into a regenerative process. Although erythropoiesis occurs in peripheral blood, the primary site of hematopoiesis in general is the kidney in teleosts and the Leydig organ, epigonal organ, thymus, and spleen in the elasmobranch.[21,22]

Packed Cell Volume

The most common diagnostic tool used to evaluate the amount of RBCs is the packed cell volume (PCV). The PCV, or hematocrit, is the concentration of RBCs per volume of blood and is expressed as a percentage. The 2 terms are used interchangeably, but the hematocrit usually represents a calculated result whereas the PCV is a direct measurement from centrifuged blood. The normal range in teleosts is approximately 20% to 45%.[19,22] The normal range in sharks is more difficult because of the significant difference in results based on venipuncture site. The PCV tends to be lower in samples collected from the venous sinus near the dorsal fin than from those collected from the caudal vein of the tail.[29,30] Other factors that may contribute to PCV variation in healthy animals include stress (handling, anesthesia, water intake), physical characteristics (size, species), sex, environmental factors (water temperature, dissolved oxygen, population density, photoperiod), activity level (thermodynamics), reproductive status, life stage, and diet. Anemia is classified as hematocrit less than 20%, and may be due to blood loss (hemorrhagic anemia), cell destruction (hemolytic anemia), or decreased production (hypoplastic anemia).[25] Polycythemia is classified as hematocrit greater than 45% and may due to dehydration, sexually mature males, hypoxia, stress, splenic contraction, or erythrocyte swelling.[25] Some of the causes for a change in the PCV are summarized in **Table 4**. There is also a summary available regarding anemia in another report.[25]

Red Blood Cell Indices

In addition to hematocrit, other measures involving the RBCs include the total count, hemoglobin, and the indices mean cell volume (MCV), mean corpuscular hemoglobin concentration (MCHC), and mean cell hemoglobin (MCH). The preferred method of determining the total RBC count is manually, as automatic blood analyzers are not able to differentiate between RBCs and white blood cells (WBCs), thereby accruing a small margin of error. Determination of both types of cell counts is done manually using two different methods (one for erythrocytes and one for leukocytes) with a hemacytometer. For both types of cell counts, the Natt-Herricks solution kit (Natt-Pette) is used for fish, as they tend to be more lymphocytic. The kit contains prefilled Natt-Herricks stain reservoirs, a pipette calibrated for 5 μL (to make the 1:200 dilution), and tips for the pipette. The following steps are taken to establish the total RBC count:

1. Draw 5 μL of blood using the pipette and tip, and wipe the tip of any excess blood with a lint free cloth or tissue.
2. Add blood to the Natt-Herricks stain reservoir and gently flush sample from the tip with the plunger of the pipette.
3. Apply a rocking motion to the reservoir to mix the sample and allow to set for at least 5 minutes.
4. Set up the hemacytometer with a specifically designed coverslip, fill each chamber with the solution using capillary action, and allow to set for 5 to 10 minutes (**Fig. 6**).
5. Using the 10× objective on the microscope, note the grid of 9 large squares. Center the large center square and adjust to the 40× objective (**Fig. 7**).

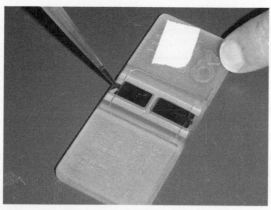

Fig. 6. The hemacytometer is loaded with a blood sample mixed with Natt-Herricks solution.

6. Count all the RBCs in the center square and 4 corner squares within the large center square. The RBCs will be elliptical cells with a centralized nucleus. The cytoplasm intensity may vary within a single sample depending on stain uptake for that particular cell (see **Fig. 7**).
7. Multiply the count for the 5 squares by 10,000 to calculate the total number of RBCs/mm^3 (or μL).

The hemoglobin concentration is typically measured using the cyanomethemoglobin method. The combination of the reagent and blood mixture should be centrifuged before measuring to remove the free nuclei.[16,19] Most teleost hemoglobin concentrations range from 5 to 10 g/dL.[19]

The MCV, MCHC, and MCH are collectively known as the RBC indices. The standard method for calculating the indices for other vertebrates can be used for fish. The equations and typical reference intervals for teleosts are shown in **Table 2**. The intervals shown are merely an estimate, as many factors may contribute to slight variation. For example, active fish will have a higher demand for oxygen and, therefore, a smaller RBC count and a lower MCV.[19,28] Elasmobranchs, in general, have larger and fewer erythrocytes that contain more hemoglobin in comparison with bony fish, which translates into increased MCV, MCHC, and MCH but decreased PCV, hemoglobin

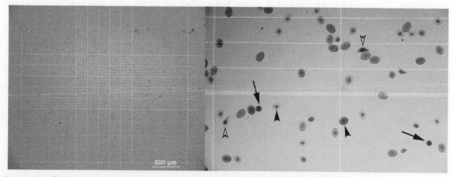

Fig. 7. (*Left*) The 9-square grid of the hemacytometer chamber. (*Right*) The hemacytometer chamber at 40× magnification for cell evaluation. The solid arrowheads indicate red blood cells. The open arrowheads indicate thrombocytes. The solid arrows indicate leukocytes. ([*Left*] *Courtesy of* Eric Carlson, BS, Denver, CO.)

Table 2
Red blood cell indices and their corresponding reference interval for teleost fish

Red Blood Cell Indices	Reference Interval for Teleosts[19]
MCV (fL) = [PCV (%) × 10]/Total RBC	150–350 fL
MCH (pg) = [Hb (g/dL) × 10]/Total RBC	30–100 pg
MCHC (g/dL) = [Hb (g/dL) × 100]/PCV (%)	18%–30% (or g/dL)

Abbreviations: Hb, hemoglobin; MCH, mean cell hemoglobin; MCHC, mean corpuscular hemoglobin concentration; MCV, mean cell volume; PCV, packed cell volume; RBC, red blood cells.

concentration, and total RBCs.[31] Similar to PCV, other factors that may contribute to changes in these values are cell maturity (the more mature, the larger the cell, thereby increasing values), species, season, and diet.

Leukocyte Structure and Function

Similar to other vertebrates, fish have granulocytes and agranulocytes, with the agranulocytes being lymphocytes and monocytes. There is warranted confusion regarding the nomenclature of fish granulocytes, owing to their apparent diversity. Some fish granulocytes have an appearance similar to that of avian (heterophil) or mammalian (neutrophil) cells, hence the adoption of those terms in some cases. Analyzing the cellular ultrastructure with the use of an electron microscope and cytochemical staining can be done to help standardize the classification of teleost granulocytes. One study showed that koi, *Cyprinus carpio*, possessed neutrophils, eosinophils, and basophils, and confirmed the presence of lymphocytes and monocytes by using electron microscopy and cytochemical staining.[32] The same study suggested that cell identification might be more effectively accomplished by using more than 1 evaluation method. An example supporting this claim is with channel catfish, *Ictalurus punctatus*. One study[33] identified these fish as having neutrophils, basophils, lymphocytes, and monocytes using both electron microscopy and cytochemical staining while another[34] declared heterophils as the primary granulocyte, using electron microscopy only. In most cases of bony fish, the predominant leukocyte will have a similar appearance to the Romanowsky-stained avian or reptile heterophil, but may have the cytochemical properties of a mammalian neutrophil. From here on the primary teleost leukocyte is referred to as a neutrophil. Neutrophils are generally round with an eccentric nucleus. The basophilic nucleus can vary in shape: round, elongated, kidney-shaped, or segmented. The cytoplasm may be clear, light blue, or gray, and filled with colorless

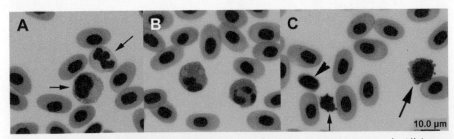

Fig. 8. Various blood cells from a white sturgeon (*Acipenser transmontanus*). All images show an abundance of red blood cells (not labeled). (*A*) Arrow on the left indicates a monocyte and arrow on the right indicates a neutrophil. (*B*) Two eosinophils. (*C*) Arrowhead indicates a thrombocyte, small arrow indicates a small lymphocyte, and large arrow indicates a large lymphocyte. Wright-Giemsa stain, 100×. (*Courtesy of* Terry Campbell, DVM, PhD, Fort Collins, CO.)

to slightly stained granules (**Fig. 8**A). Neutrophils play a primary role in the inflammatory process. In most species, neutrophils are involved with phagocytosis, but the time at which it occurs with respect to the initial insult and the duration varies among species.[35]

Eosinophils in bony fish are rare, but when seen are of similar size to slightly larger than the neutrophil, round with a round or lobed basophilic nucleus, and eosinophilic granules (see **Fig. 8**B). The cytoplasm is often a pale blue color. Eosinophils can be involved the defense against parasite infestation; however, fish that do not possess eosinophils rely on other cells to facilitate in this role.[35]

Basophils are also rare in teleosts but have been reported in some species.[18,35] Basophils are small, round cells with basophilic granules and nucleus. Many times the granules are so densely packed in the cytoplasm that the nucleus is difficult to see.

In elasmobranchs, the same apparent leukocytes exist; however, the discrepancy is not necessarily between whether a particular cell is a heterophil or neutrophil, but rather the term associated with that cell. Moreover, a single species may contain both types. The leukocytes of elasmobranchs have been determined to be G_1 (also referred to as type I, heterophil, and fine eosinophilic granulocyte or FEG), G_2 (also referred to as type II and neutrophil), and G_3 (also referred to as type III, eosinophil, and coarse eosinophilic granulocyte or CEG). It is likely species dependent, but these 3 cell types are similar in size.[30,36] The G_1 cell is usually round with an eccentric and round, indented, or segmented nucleus with fine eosinophilic granules (**Fig. 9**A). When evaluating the blood film of elasmobranchs, leukocytes that may have segmented or nonsegmented nuclei may contain both types, and should be recognized as the same cell. The G_2 cell is often round with an eccentric and round, indented, or segmented nucleus and indistinct granules. The granules and margin or the cell are often difficult to view and can be easily overlooked (see **Fig. 9**C). The G_3 cell is also typically round with a round nucleus and relatively large, round eosinophilic granules (see **Fig. 9**). This cell is often referred to as an eosinophil, but compared with bony fish is more commonly seen in elasmobranchs. Basophils may occasionally be found in the

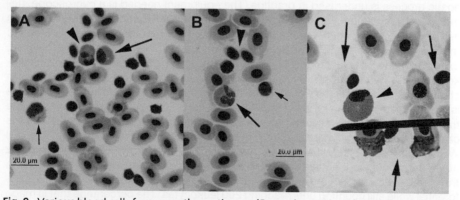

Fig. 9. Various blood cells from a southern stingray (*Dasyatis americana*). All images show an abundance of red blood cells in addition to several lymphocytes and thrombocytes (not labeled). (*A*) Large arrow indicates a G_1 (heterophil) cell, arrowhead indicates a G_3 (eosinophil) cell, and small arrow indicates a monocyte. (*B*) Large arrow indicates a segmented G_1 (heterophil) cell, small arrow indicates a lymphocyte, and arrowhead indicates 2 thrombocytes. (*C*) Large arrows indicate G_2 (neutrophils) cells; arrowhead indicates a G_1 (heterophil) cell. Wright-Giemsa stain, 100×.

peripheral blood of elasmobranchs, appearing as round cells with dark purple-stained granules. The amount of granules varies from sparse to obliterating the nucleus.

The lymphocytes and monocytes of teleosts and elasmobranchs are the most abundant cell type,[19,21,24] and have an appearance similar to that of lymphocytes of other vertebrates. Lymphocytes are occasionally described by size (small, medium, large), with the smaller cells being more mature and allowing the nucleus to occupy more cytoplasmic "real estate."[21] Combinations of different sizes may appear in one sample. Small lymphocytes are the most commonly seen in the peripheral blood of fish, being usually round with a high nucleus to cytoplasm ratio (see **Figs. 8**C and **9**B). The nucleus is round and contains dark basophilic chromatin. The cytoplasm is dark blue, occupying the occasional smooth but often irregular margins of the cell. This cell may also conform to the shape of the cells surrounding it.

Monocytes, as with other animals, are the largest leukocyte found in the peripheral blood of fish. Their shape varies from round to amoeba-like with a large, round to kidney-shaped basophilic nucleus. The cytoplasm is usually blue and may present with vacuoles (see **Figs. 8**A and **9**A). Fish monocytes also migrate into the tissue, where they are referred to as macrophages. The term macrophage is occasionally used to describe monocytes in fish because the appearance of the cell is similar to its stages during the migration into the tissue.[22]

Thrombocytes

Thrombocytes in fish are similar to mammalian platelets, and are important in the coagulation process and clot formation. Thrombocytes vary in shape among the species, but generally are round to elliptical and have a centrally positioned nucleus. The cytoplasm is usually clear but may have occasional, sparse, slightly eosinophilic granules, in which case they may be referred to as reactive. The cell margins are usually smooth, but cell clumping can also be seen (see **Figs. 8**C and **9**B).

Complete Blood Count (Hemacytometer)

As previously mentioned, the preferred method for establishing the total WBC count is by a manual method. This relatively easy, inexpensive, and potentially valuable diagnostic process is underused in practice. The equipment needed is a microscope, hemacytometer, counter, and the Natt-Herricks kit (the Natt-Herricks solution is used in fish because of their abundance of lymphocytes). To determine the total WBC count, the steps for determining the RBC count through step 5 listed earlier are followed, except that advancement to the 40× objective may not be necessary. Next, all the leukocytes with or without the thrombocytes in all 9 large squares of the grid in both chambers are counted (see **Fig. 7**). If the difference between counts in both chambers is greater than 10%, the process should be repeated. It is challenging to discern the thrombocytes from leukocytes; therefore, including them can be adjusted for in the calculation after the differential is performed. If only the leukocytes are counted, a total WBC count can be immediately calculated using the equation: WBC count/mm^3 (or μL) = (total count in 9 squares + 10%) × 200.[16] If the thrombocytes are included in the count, the thrombocytes are counted independent of the leukocytes during the differential while still counting until reaching 200 leukocytes. The percentage that is made up by the thrombocytes is then subtracted from the hemacytometer count.[19] The reference intervals for fish leukocytes varies, and normal variations from those respective intervals may occur based on species, season (water temperature), age, sex, diet, or stress. Reference intervals for select teleosts and elasmobranchs are shown in **Tables 3** and **4**. Because the basophil counts are low for both types of fish, they are not included in the tables.

Blood Smear and Differential

A blood smear can provide a wealth of information; therefore, even if only a drop of blood is collected, it should not go to waste. The blood smear is evaluated after processing the slide through any Romanowsky stain, which helps to visualize and identify different cell types. Viewing the slide at low power initially can subjectively offer an idea of cell type distribution, which is especially useful information if insufficient blood has been collected for a complete blood count. At higher power, the cells can be evaluated more closely. Owing to the diversity of fish and, consequently, their cells, it is recommended to scan over the slide initially to see which cells are present and to check the quality of the smear. Once a comfort level is established among cell types, the differential can be more effectively performed. Each cell is counted individually until a total leukocyte count of 200 is reached. The percentage of each cell type is used to calculate the absolute number using the total leukocyte count obtained from the hemacytometer.

Morphologic evaluation of the cells and identifying any inclusions, toxicity, polychromasia (noted by the presence of immature cells), pathogens, or artifacts should also be performed when viewing the blood smear. Toxic changes to neutrophils or heterophils appear during systemic illness and may aid with prognosis (**Fig. 10**). The degree of toxicity should be noted, because the greater the number of toxic cells present, the poorer the prognosis.[22] Intracellular or extracellular parasites may be present. For example, apicomplexan hemoparasites may be seen in the cytoplasm of RBCs (**Fig. 11**).[46,49] Depending on the history of the animal's health and the environmental conditions, some parasites may be incidental findings or contribute to alterations in cell counts (anemia, eosinophilia). Viral diseases represent another disorder that may alter the cell morphology whereby a blood smear evaluation would contribute to the diagnosis. Several diseases have been reported in which intracellular inclusions have been observed, such as viral erythrocytic necrosis, erythrocytic inclusion body syndrome, and intraerythrocytic viral disease.[49] The quality of the blood smear preparation or anticoagulant may negatively affect the cells. Often in an aquatic environment, humidity or water contamination can affect the preparation or the cell architecture. Certain anticoagulants may also affect the cells. For example, Na$_2$EDTA has been reported as inducing RBC swelling, anisocytosis, anisonucleosis, and hemolysis.[20]

Interpretation of Results

Although there is a growing database of reference intervals and information regarding cellular ultrastructure and chemistry, interpreting the results can be difficult. Some strategies to overcome this challenge may be to extrapolate from a similar species with known information, collect a sample from a tank mate of the same species to use as a control, extrapolate from general knowledge, or plan on collecting sequential samples to analyze the trend in a particular fish. **Tables 3** and **4** provide a summary of publications with established reference intervals for particular species. There are also publications that provide extensive tables with reference values.[19,31] Regardless, the interpretation is difficult because the functionality of many cell types is still uncertain.

Table 5 summarizes reports of intrinsic and extrinsic factors that affect hematologic parameters, and the direction (increased or decreased) in which they were affected. Many of the disease conditions affecting PCV that cause anemia have been described,[25] and therefore are not repeated here. In cases of anemia, fish are treated similarly to other animals. Blood transfusion is an option that has been reported on occasion. Elasmobranchs of the same species had no reaction to transfusion,[66] and

Table 3
Reference intervals for erythrocyte parameters of select teleosts and elasmobranchs

	PCV (%)	RBC (×10⁶/µL)	Hb (g/dL)	MCV (fL)	MCH (pg)	MCHC (g/dL)
Teleosts						
Acipenser brevirostrum Shortnose sturgeon[37]	26–46	0.65–1.09	5.7–8.7	307–520	65.9–107.1	15–30
Acipenser fulvescens Wild Lake Sturgeon[38]	17–38	—	—	—	—	—
Carassius auratus Goldfish[18]	21.3–23.3	0.8–2.4	6.45–6.95	134.4–139.6	40.6–43.4	0.3
Cichlasoma dimerus South American cichlid[39]	22.5–39.12	1.68–4.27	5.23–8.33	70.14–198	14.51–40.59	17.43–30.31
Colossoma brachypomum Red pacu[40]	20–32	0.98–2.95	—	—	—	—
Cyprinus carpio Common koi carp[18,32]	31.9–34.9	1.59–1.75	7.84–8.56	196.5–207.5	49.1	0.24
Ictalurus punctatus Farmed channel catfish[41]	27–54	1.5–4.1	4.4–10.9	88.6–186.7	—	15.7–28.7
Lutjanus guttatus Spotted rose snapper[42]	33.53–71.14	0.75–3.71	7.29–17.03	135.66–369.80	20.1–91.47	11.16–31.09
Oreochromis hybrid Tilapia[43]	27–37	1.91–2.83	7.0–9.8	115–183	28.3–42.3	22–29
Pterois volitans Red lion fish[44]	27–44	—	—	—	—	—
Elasmobranchs						
Alopias vulpinus Common thresher[45]	28.5–46.4	—	11.2–16.1	—	—	34.3–39.3
Carcharhinus obscurus Dusky shark[45]	9.4–25	—	3.1–8.7	—	—	32.4–38

Species				
Carcharhinus plumbeus Sandbar shark[36,45]	9.4–24	—	3.2–8.4	25.7–41.2
Carcharodon carcharias Great white shark[45]	22–49	—	8.2–16.2	31.2–43.1
Dasyatis americana Captive southern stingrays[46]	21–36	—	—	—
Galeocerdo cuvieri Tiger shark[45]	9.4–33	—	3.2–10.1	27.9–40
Isurus oxyrinchus Atlantic shortfin mako[45]	22.5–60	—	9.6–21.1	33.1–41.1
Mustelus canis Smooth dogfish[47]	20.1–28.3 (F) 27.3–32.1 (M)	—	—	—
Prionace glauca Blue shark[45]	9.4–22.5	—	3.1–7.6	27.9–40.4
Rhinoptera bonasus Captive cownose stingray[47]	27–35	0.38–0.54	—	—
Rhizoprionodon terraenovae Atlantic sharpnose[48]	18.9–30.8	—	—	—
Squalus acanthias Spiny dogfish[48]	15–22.8	—	—	—
Sphyrna lewini Scalloped hammerhead shark[45]	26.5	—	10	37.7
Sphyrna tiburo Bonnethead shark[48]	22–35	—	—	—

Hrubec and Smith[19] provide a list of additional teleosts, and Filho et al[31] provide a comparative study of 80 different marine teleosts and elasmobranchs.
Abbreviations: F, female; M, male.

Table 4
Reference intervals for leukocyte parameters of select teleosts and elasmobranchs

	WBC ($\times 10^3$/μL)	Heterophil ($\times 10^3$/μL)	Neutrophil ($\times 10^3$/μL)	Eosinophil ($\times 10^3$/μL)	Lymphocyte ($\times 10^3$/μL)	Monocytes ($\times 10^3$/μL)
Teleosts						
Acipenser brevirostrum Shortnose sturgeon[37]	28.4–90.8	—	3.8–33.6	0–1.5	9.1–56.7 (sm) 2.1–10.4 (lg)	0–7.1
Acipenser fulvescens Wild lake sturgeon[38]	2.7–23.2	—	0.2–6.1	0–0.6	1.4–14.0	0.1–1.7
Carassius auratus Goldfish[18]	47.4–57.2	—	1.74–2.86	0.0–0.2	23.1–29.6	0.1–0.3
Cichlasoma dimerus South American cichlid[39]	6.64–18.59	1.87–5.24	—	1.02–2.85	2.55–7.14	1.19–3.34
Colossoma brachypomum Red pacu[40]	13.5–57.5	0.2–19.1	—	0.13–0.3	7.8–35.9	0.38–0.518
Cyprinus carpio Common koi carp[18,32]	34.9–40.7*	—	3%–10%	0.5%–1%	88%–93%	0.5%–2.0%
Lutjanus guttatus Spotted rose snapper[42]	25.19–111.22	—	0.19%–8.40%	0.64%–7.8%	82.58%–100%	0.55%–5.37%
Oreochromis hybrid Tilapia[43]	21.56–154.69	—	0.56–9.87	0.04–1.65	6.78–136.4 (sm) 2.85–30.8 (lg)	0.4–4.29
Pterois volitans Red lion fish[44]	2.0–8.2	13%–72%	—	—	7%–67%	16%–51%

Elasmobranchs

Dasyatis americana Captive southern stingray[46]	3.8–27.9	1.0–8.9	0.1–3.1	0–0.9	1.1–30.1	0–1.0
Mustelus canis Smooth dogfish[47]	11.24–19.42 (F) 7.86–20.74 (M)	2.37–8.21 (F) 1.57–4.69 (M)	2.33–4.41 (F) 2.06–4.69 (M)	0.28–0.92 (F) 0.4–1.28 (M)	3.08–6.74 (F) 1.69–8.87 (M)	0.42–1.91 (F) 0.6–2.75 (M)
Rhincodon typus Captive whale shark[30]	5.09	2.01	0.05	0.33	2.37	0.32
Rhinoptera bonasus Captive cownose stingray[47]	0.17–1.98	0–72 (seg) 0–55 (non)	—	0–77 (seg) 0–83 (non)	0.14–1.88	0–26
Rhizoprionodon terraenovae Atlantic sharpnose[45]	34.6–119.6	5.7–26.8	0.0–2.6	2.2–22.7	10.4–47.4	0.0–6.5
Squalus acanthias Spiny dogfish[48]	21.4–55.9	2.0–11.2	1.3–18.2	1.1–11.4	7.6–23.4	0.41–3.3
Sphyrna tiburo Bonnethead shark[48]	35.3–83.1	4.7–19.1	6.7–8.5	0.34–12.1	10.4–37.5	0.47–4.6

Hrubec and Smith[19] provide a list of additional teleosts, and Filho et al[31] provide a comparative study of 80 different marine teleosts and elasmobranchs.

Abbreviations: F, female; lg, large; M, male; non, nonsegmented; seg, segmented; sm, small.

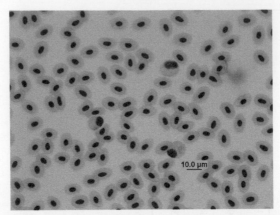

Fig. 10. An example of toxic neutrophils in a koi (*Cyprinus carpio*). Wright-Giemsa stain, 100×. (*Courtesy of* Terry Campbell, DVM, PhD, Fort Collins, CO.)

similar success has been documented in teleosts within the same taxonomic group[67]; however, cross-matching is recommended. Of course, similar conditions and diseases will also affect the other erythrocyte parameters. Hemoglobin is elevated in endothermic sharks in comparison with ectothermic sharks,[45] induced starvation,[53] and elasmobranchs in comparison with teleosts,[31] and is decreased in trout (*Oncorhynchus mykiss*) with viral hemorrhagic septicemia (VHS)[50] and in common carp (*C carpio*) with *Aeromonas* infection.[54] Similarly, the RBC indices also increased with induced starvation in traíra (*Hoplias malabaricus*)[53] and decreased with VHS in trout (*O mykiss*).[50]

The factors affecting leukocyte count are also represented in **Table 5**. In general, a stress leukogram is often defined as a relative leukocytosis with a lymphopenia. Elevated leukocytes as a result of a neutrophilia or heterophilia may also be associated with an inflammatory disease, although the actual function of such cells is unclear. Various disease processes have shown changes in total WBC count from low to high or high to low during different stages of the disease or severity of the insult. For example, channel catfish (*I punctatus*) showed a decrease in total WBC count when fed lower concentrations of *Fusarium moniliforme*, and increased counts

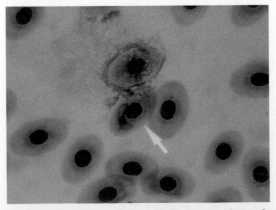

Fig. 11. *Light green arrow*: Hemogregarine parasite in the cytoplasm of a red blood cell in a southern stingray, *Dasyatis americana*. Diff Quik stain, 100×.

Table 5
Summary of some intrinsic and extrinsic factors that affect primary hematologic parameters

Parameter	Increased	Decreased
PCV	Stress: splenic contraction[16] Capture stress or inadequate anesthesia inducing RBC swelling[19] Male vs female smooth dogfish[51] Endothermic vs ectothermic sharks[45] Teleosts > sharks > rays[21,31] Increased activity level[21,31] Exposure to herbicide[56] Dactylogyrid monogenean infestation[42] Coccidiosis in carp[59]	Stress: increased water intake[16] VHS in trout[50] Younger fish[52] Starvation in traira[53] Dietary *Fusarium moniliforme*[54] Southern stingray in tourists sites (diet, parasites, crowding)[55] Sea louse infection in trout[57] *Aeromonas* infection in carp[58]
Hemoglobin	Endothermic vs ectothermic sharks[45] Induced starvation[53] Elasmobranchs vs teleosts[31]	VHS in trout[50] *Aeromonas* infection in carp[58]
RBC count	Coccidiosis in carp[59] Summer seasons in trout[60]	VHS in trout[50] Dietary *Fusarium moniliforme*[54] Sea louse infection in trout[57] *Aeromonas* infection in carp[58] Induced starvation[53]
MCV	Induced starvation[53]	VHS in trout[50]
MCHC	Induced starvation[53]	VHS in trout[50]
Total WBC count	Spring and summer seasons[61] Young fish[52] Stress[25] *Aeromonas hydrophila* injection[58] Higher concentrations of dietary *Fusarium moniliforme*[54] Dactylogyrid monogenean infestation[42] Exposure to herbicide[56] Zinc exposure[65] Traumatic clasper lesions[37]	Autumn and winter seasons[60] In low temperatures[62] Induced starvation[53] Stress (confinement, low water, chasing, netting)[63] Lower concentrations of dietary *Fusarium moniliforme*[54] Acute copper exposure[64]
Heterophils/ neutrophils	Day 8 coccidiosis infection[59] Female vs male[51] (FEG, CEG) Chronic copper exposure[64]	Initial (day 5) coccidiosis infection[59]
Eosinophils	Dactylogyrid monogenean infestation[60]	
Monocytes	Day 8 coccidiosis infection[59]	Initial (day 5) coccidiosis infection[59]
Lymphocytes	Initial (day 5) coccidiosis infection[59]	Day 8 coccidiosis infection[59] Stress[25] Sea louse infection in trout (stress or increased cortisol)[57] Chronic copper exposure[64]
Thrombocytes	Dactylogyrid monogenean infestation[42] Chronic copper exposure[64]	

Abbreviations: CEG, G$_3$ leukocytes (coarse eosinophilic granulocyte); FEG, G$_1$ leukocytes (fine eosinophilic granulocyte); VHS, viral hemorrhagic septicemia; WBC, white blood cells.

when fed high concentrations of the fungal toxins.[54] Another study showed an increase in leukocytes in common carp after 10 days of being infected with an *Aeromonas hydrophila* injection.[58] The leukocyte count continued to increase through the 30th day of the infected fish, whereas the leukocyte count of treated fish came down after the 10th day. Carp infected with a coccidian (*Goussia carpelli*) initially (by day 5) showed an increase in lymphocytes and a decrease in granulocytes and monocytes, but showed opposite results by day 8.[59] White-spotted bamboo sharks (*Chiloscyllium plagiosum*) with traumatic clasper lesions had increased total WBC counts as a result of heterophilia when compared with their tank mates without lesions (Carlson E. White-spotted bamboo sharks [*Chiloscyllium plagiosum*]: clasper removal and hematology findings. Unpublished data presented at the Regional Aquatics Workshop, 2012). As a potential treatment option, the claspers of the affected sharks were removed, and subsequently the WBC counts returned to their presumed normal range. There are many other documented disease processes that presumably affect WBC counts, some of which are presented in **Table 5**.

REFERENCES

1. Available at: https://www.flmnh.ufl.edu/fish/education/questions/questions.html. Accessed July 27, 2014.
2. Claver JA, Quaglia AI. Comparative morphology, development, and function of blood cells in nonmammalian vertebrates. Journal of Exotic Pet Medicine 2009; 18(2):87–97.
3. Available at: http://www.petplace.com/dogs/how-many-pets-are-in-the-us/page1.aspx. Accessed July 14, 2014.
4. Roberts HE. Physical examination of fish. In: Roberts HE, editor. Fundamentals of ornamental fish health. Ames (IA): John Wiley & Sons; 2010. p. 161–5.
5. Dyer SM, Cervasio EL. An overview of restraint and blood collection techniques in exotic pet practice. Vet Clin North Am Exot Anim Pract 2008;11(3):423–43.
6. Ross LG. Restraint, anaesthesia and euthanasia. In: Wildgoose WH, editor. BSAVA manual of ornamental fish. Gloucester (United Kingdom): British Small Animal Veterinary Association; 2001. p. 75–89.
7. Brooks EJ, Sloman KA, Liss S, et al. The stress physiology of extended duration tonic immobility in the juvenile lemon shark, *Negaprion brevirostris* (Poey 1868). J Exp Mar Bio Ecol 2011;409(1):351–60.
8. Henningsen AD. Tonic immobility in 12 elasmobranchs: use as an aid in captive husbandry. Zoo Biol 1994;13(4):325–32.
9. Watsky MA, Gruber SH. Induction and duration of tonic immobility in the lemon shark, *Negaprion brevirostris*. Fish Physiol Biochem 1990;8(3):207–10.
10. Stamper MA. Elasmobranchs (sharks, rays, and skates). In: West G, Heard D, Caulkett N, editors. Zoo animal and wildlife immobilization and anesthesia. Ames (IA): Blackwell Publishing; 2007. p. 197–203.
11. Carter KM, Woodley CM, Brown RS. A review of tricaine methanesulfonate for anesthesia of fish. Reviews in Fish Biology and Fisheries 2011;21(1):51–9.
12. Neiffer DL, Stamper MA. Fish sedation, anesthesia, analgesia, and euthanasia: considerations, methods, and types of drugs. ILAR J 2009;50(4):343–60.
13. Neiffer DL. Boney fish (lungfish, sturgeon, and teleosts). In: West G, Heard D, Caulkett N, editors. Zoo animal and wildlife immobilization and anesthesia. Ames (IA): Blackwell Publishing; 2007. p. 147–266.
14. Sneddon LU. Clinical anesthesia and analgesia in fish. Journal of Exotic Pet Medicine 2012;21(1):32–43.

15. Roberts HE. Anesthesia, analgesia, and euthanasia. In: Roberts HE, editor. Fundamentals of ornamental fish health. Ames (IA): John Wiley & Sons; 2010. p. 166–71.
16. Campbell TW, Ellis CK. Avian and exotic animal hematology and cytology. Ames (IA): John Wiley & Sons; 2007.
17. Roberts HE, Weber SE, Smith SA. Nonlethal diagnostic techniques. In: Roberts HE, editor. Fundamentals of ornamental fish health. Ames (IA): John Wiley & Sons; 2010. p. 172–84.
18. Groff JM, Zinkl JG. Hematology and clinical chemistry of cyprinid fish. Common carp and goldfish. Vet Clin North Am Exot Anim Pract 1999;2(3):741–76.
19. Hrubec TC, Smith SA. Hematology of fishes. In: Weiss DJ, Wardrop KJ, editors. Schalm's veterinary hematology. Ames (IA): John Wiley & Sons; 2010. p. 994–1003.
20. Walencik J, Witeska M. The effects of anticoagulants on hematological indices and blood cell morphology of common carp (*Cyprinus carpio* L.). Comp Biochem Physiol C Toxicol Pharmacol 2007;146(3):331–5.
21. Walsh CJ, Luer CA. Elasmobranch hematology. In: Warmolts D, Thoney D, Hueter R, editors. The elasmobranch husbandry manual: captive care of sharks, rays and their relatives. Columbus (OH): Ohio Biological Survey; 2004. p. 301–23.
22. Fánge R. Fish blood cells. Fish Physiol 1992;12:1–54.
23. Wingstrand KG. Nonnucleated erythrocytes in a teleostean fish *Maurolicus mülleri* (Gmelin). Z Zellforsch Mikrosk Anat 1956;45(2):195–200.
24. Campbell TW. Hematology of fish. In: Thrall MA, Weiser G, Allison R, et al, editors. Veterinary hematology and clinical chemistry. Ames (IA): John Wiley & Sons; 2012. p. 298–312.
25. Clauss TM, Dove AD, Arnold JE. Hematologic disorders of fish. Vet Clin North Am Exot Anim Pract 2008;11(3):445–62.
26. Available at: http://www.genomesize.com/cellsize/fish.htm. Accessed July 31, 2014.
27. Gregory TR. The bigger the C-value, the larger the cell: genome size and red blood cell size in vertebrates. Blood Cells Mol Dis 2001;27(5):830–43.
28. Maciak S, Janko K, Kotusz J, et al. Standard metabolic rate (SMR) is inversely related to erythrocyte and genome size in allopolyploid fish of the *Cobitis taenia* hybrid complex. Functional Ecology 2011;25(5):1072–8.
29. Mylniczenko ND, Curtis EW, Wilborn RE, et al. Differences in hematocrit of blood samples obtained from 2 venipuncture sites in sharks. Am J Vet Res 2006;67(11): 1861–4.
30. Dove AD, Arnold J, Clauss TM. Blood cells and serum chemistry in the world's largest fish: the whale shark *Rhincodon typus*. Aquatic Biology 2010;9(2):177–83.
31. Filho DW, Eble GJ, Kassner G, et al. Comparative hematology in marine fish. Comp Biochem Physiol Comp Physiol 1992;102(2):311–21.
32. Tripathi NK, Latimer KS, Burnley VV. Hematologic reference intervals for koi (*Cyprinus carpio*), including blood cell morphology, cytochemistry, and ultrastructure. Vet Clin Pathol 2004;33(2):74–83.
33. Tavares-Dias M, Moraes FR. Leukocyte and thrombocyte reference values for channel catfish (*Ictalurus punctatus* Raf), with an assessment of morphologic, cytochemical, and ultrastructural features. Vet Clin Pathol 2007;36(1):49–54.
34. Cannon MS, Mollenhauer HH, Eurell TE, et al. An ultrastructural study of the leukocytes of the channel catfish, Ictalurus punctatus. J Morphol 1980;164(1):1–23.
35. Ainsworth AJ. Fish granulocytes: morphology, distribution, and function. Annual Review of Fish Diseases 1992;2:123–48.

36. Arnold JE. Hematology of the sandbar shark, *Carcharhinus plumbeus*: standardization of complete blood count techniques for elasmobranchs. Vet Clin Pathol 2005;34(2):115–23.

37. Knowles S, Hrubec TC, Smith SA, et al. Hematology and plasma chemistry reference intervals for cultured shortnose sturgeon (*Acipenser brevirostrum*). Vet Clin Pathol 2006;35(4):434–40.

38. DiVincenti L, Wyatt J, Priest H, et al. Reference intervals for select hematologic and plasma biochemical analytes of wild Lake Sturgeon (*Acipenser fulvescens*) from the St. Lawrence River in New York. Vet Clin Pathol 2013;42(1):19–26.

39. Rey Vázquez G, Guerrero GA. Characterization of blood cells and hematological parameters in *Cichlasoma dimerus* (Teleostei, Perciformes). Tissue Cell 2007; 39(3):151–60.

40. Tocidlowski ME, Lewbart GA, Stoskopf MK. Hematologic study of red pacu (*Colossoma brachypomum*). Vet Clin Pathol 1997;26(3):119–25.

41. Tavares-Dias M, Moraes FR. Haematological and biochemical reference intervals for farmed channel catfish. J Fish Biol 2007;71(2):383–8.

42. Del Rio-Zaragoza OB, Fajer-Ávila EJ, Almazán-Rueda P, et al. Hematological characteristics of the spotted rose snapper *Lutjanus guttatus* (Steindachner, 1869) healthy and naturally infected by dactylogyrid monogeneans. Tissue Cell 2011;43(3):137–42.

43. Hrubec TC, Cardinale JL, Smith SA. Hematology and plasma chemistry reference intervals for cultured tilapia (*Oreochromis hybrid*). Vet Clin Pathol 2000;29(1): 7–12.

44. Anderson ET, Stoskopf MK, Morris JA Jr, et al. Hematology, plasma biochemistry, and tissue enzyme activities of invasive red lionfish captured off North Carolina, USA. J Aquat Anim Health 2010;22(4):266–73.

45. Emery SH. Hematological comparisons of endothermic vs ectothermic elasmobranch fishes. Copeia 1986;1986(3):700–5.

46. Campbell TW, Grant KR. Clinical cases in avian & exotic animal hematology & cytology. Ames (IA): Wiley-Blackwell; 2010.

47. Ferreira CM, Field CL, Tuttle AD. Hematological and plasma biochemical parameters of aquarium-maintained cownose rays. J Aquat Anim Health 2010;22(2): 123–8.

48. Haman KH, Norton TM, Thomas AC, et al. Baseline health parameters and species comparisons among free-ranging Atlantic sharpnose (*Rhizoprionodon terraenovae*), bonnethead (*Sphyrna tiburo*), and spiny dogfish (*Squalus acanthias*) sharks in Georgia, Florida, and Washington, USA. J Wildl Dis 2012; 48(2):295–306.

49. Noga EJ. Fish disease: diagnosis and treatment. Ames (IA): John Wiley & Sons; 2010.

50. Rehulka J. Haematological analyses in rainbow trout *Oncorhynchus mykiss* affected by viral haemorrhagic septicaemia (VHS). Dis Aquat organ 2003; 56(3):185–93.

51. Persky ME, Williams JJ, Burks RE, et al. Hematologic, plasma biochemistry, and select nutrient values in captive smooth dogfish (*Mustelus canis*). J Zoo Wildl Med 2012;43(4):842–51.

52. Hrubec TC, Smith SA, Robertson JL. Age-related changes in hematology and plasma chemistry values of hybrid striped bass (*Morone chrysops* × *Morone saxatilis*). Vet Clin Pathol 2001;30(1):8–15.

53. Rios FS, Oba ET, Fernandes MN, et al. Erythrocyte senescence and haematological changes induced by starvation in the neotropical fish traíra, *Hoplias*

malabaricus (Characiformes, Erythrinidae). Comp Biochem Physiol A Mol Integr Physiol 2005;140(3):281–7.

54. Lumlertdacha S, Lovell RT, Shelby RA, et al. Growth, hematology, and histopathology of channel catfish, *Ictalurus punctatus*, fed toxins from *Fusarium moniliforme*. Aquaculture 1995;130(2):201–18.

55. Semeniuk CA, Bourgeon S, Smith SL, et al. Hematological differences between stingrays at tourist and nonvisited sites suggest physiologic costs of wildlife tourism. Biologic Conservation 2009;142(8):1818–29.

56. Modesto KA, Martinez CB. Effects of Roundup Transorb on fish: hematology, antioxidant defenses and acetylcholinesterase activity. Chemosphere 2010;81(6): 781–7.

57. Ruane NM, Nolan DT, Rotllant J, et al. Experimental exposure of rainbow trout *Oncorhynchus mykiss* (Walbaum) to the infective stages of the sea louse *Lepeophtheirus salmonis* (Krøyer) influences the physiologic response to an acute stressor. Fish Shellfish Immunol 2000;10(5):451–63.

58. Harikrishnan R, Nisha Rani M, Balasundaram C. Hematological and biochemical parameters in common carp, *Cyprinus carpio*, following herbal treatment of *Aeromonas hydrophila* infection. Aquaculture 2003;221(1):41–50.

59. Steinhagen D, Oesterreich B, Körting W. Carp coccidiosis: clinical and hematological observations of carp infected with *Goussia carpelli*. Dis Aquat organ 1997;30:137–43.

60. Morgan AL, Thompson KD, Auchinachie NA, et al. The effect of seasonality on normal haematological and innate immune parameters of rainbow trout *Oncorhynchus mykiss* L. Fish Shellfish Immunol 2008;25(6):791–9.

61. Houston AH, Dobric N, Kahurananga R. The nature of hematological response in fish. Fish Physiol Biochem 1996;15(4):339–47.

62. Sala-Rabanal M, Sánchez J, Ibarz A, et al. Effects of low temperatures and fasting on hematology and plasma composition of gilthead sea bream (*Sparus aurata*). Fish Physiol Biochem 2003;29(2):105–15.

63. Schreck CB, Contreras-Sanchez W, Fitzpatrick MS. Fffects of stress on fish reproduction, gamete quality, and progeny. Aquaculture 2001;197(1):3–24.

64. Dick PT, Dixon DG. Changes in circulating blood cell levels of rainbow trout, *Salmo gairdneri* Richardson, following acute and chronic exposure to copper. J Fish Biol 1985;26(4):475–81.

65. Flos R, Tort L, Balasch J. Effects of zinc sulphate on haematological parameters in the dogfish, *Scyliorhinus canicula*, and influences of MS222. Mar Environ Res 1987;21(4):289–98.

66. Hadfield CA, Haines AN, Clayton LA, et al. Cross matching of blood in carcharhiniform, lamniform, and orectolobiform sharks. J Zoo Wildl Med 2010;41(3): 480–6.

67. Sakai DK, Okada H, Koide N, et al. Blood type compatibility of lower vertebrates: phylogenetic diversity in blood transfusion between fish species. Dev Comp Immunol 1988;11(1):105–15.

Reference Intervals in Avian and Exotic Hematology

Carolyn Cray, PhD

KEYWORDS

- Reference interval • Hematology • Indirect method • Index of individuality
- Biological variation

KEY POINTS

- Reference intervals are of key value in result interpretation, but interval generation is fraught with difficulties, especially in sample size, in avian and exotic medicine.
- Reference interval generation should be a systematic process, with recognition of reference population definition, sample handling, method standardization, and the use of valid statistical methods.
- Although best sample size should be met whenever possible, alternative statistical methods are viable options to generate working intervals.

INTRODUCTION

Reference data form the basis for the interpretation of health data that are collected during clinical examination and laboratory testing. In the decision process of reviewing laboratory-derived patient data, simple comparisons with data from a known normal population can provide valuable information to formulate a diagnosis or prognosis. These comparative data have been referred to as normal values and reference ranges, but the term reference interval (RI) has been adopted. The goal of the RI is to represent the most common population(s) and, in reference to veterinary medicine, to be reflective of the many species that are seen in clinical practice.

The generation of RI for avian and exotic species is especially difficult, given limitations in sample size. This difficulty is related not only to having proper access to an appropriate number of specimens but also to time and cost considerations. Recent recommendations by the American Society of Veterinary Clinical Pathology (ASVCP) provide allowances for sample sets of 20 or 40 samples in addition to the preferred

Disclosure statement: the author has nothing to disclose.
Division of Comparative Pathology, Department of Pathology, University of Miami Miller School of Medicine, PO Box 016960 (R-46), Miami, FL 33101, USA
E-mail address: ccray@med.miami.edu

Vet Clin Exot Anim 18 (2015) 105–116
http://dx.doi.org/10.1016/j.cvex.2014.09.006
1094-9194/15/$ – see front matter © 2015 Elsevier Inc. All rights reserved.

standard of n≥120.[1] These and other methods can be viable alternatives that can be used to begin to address the need for RI in avian and exotic species. Because most published intervals or values for special species do not begin to meet the important criteria, it is critical that investigators, clinicians, and publishers/editors be aware of these guidelines to move this process forward.

INFLUENCES ON REFERENCE INTERVAL GENERATION

The process of RI generation must acknowledge the potential strong influences of the population from which the samples are derived and the preanalytical and analytical procedures that are used in RI development (**Table 1**).

Reference Population Demographics

Age

Age-related changes in RI were well documented in 1-month-old to 3-month-old macaws, eclectus parrots, and cockatoos, in which total white blood cell counts were observed to decrease with age.[2–4] In a longitudinal analysis of repeated measures on a group of captive bald eagles over a 12-year period,[5] significant increases were reported for total red blood cells and percent heterophils with age. A higher total white blood cell count and lower packed cell volume was observed in young California condors[6]; the investigators recommended the use of 1 set of intervals to 6 months of age and a second interval for the subadult/adult birds. Compared with adults, the blood of 2-month-old to 3-month-old Chilean flamingos was reported to have lower red blood cell counts and packed cell volume and higher total white blood cell counts.[7] Values for red cell parameters were also found to be age related in mute swans, vinaceous Amazon parrots, and red-capped parrots.[8,9] Changes in loggerhead sea turtle hematology between the ages of 8 months and 56 months were also reported.[10] This study included a lower packed cell volume, total white blood cell count, and higher eosinophil counts in young animals; higher monocyte counts were observed in older animals. In another study of box turtles, a negative correlation between body weight and packed cell volume was reported.[11]

Species and breed

Significant differences have been reported in clinical chemistry parameters in different crossbreeds of budgerigars, although supportive data were sparse.[12] Unique intervals were also reported in an extended study of several species of macaws, cockatoos,

Table 1 Influences of RI generation	
Patient Demographics	**Preanalytical and Analytical Procedures**
Age	Fasting
Sex	Stress/travel
Exercise	Time of day
Diet	Anticoagulant
Husbandry	Specimen handling
Location	Specimen transport
Season	Defined time before analysis
Altitude	Analytical error
Species/subspecies	Maintain analytical procedures

and other psittacines, and this concept is generally accepted at the reference laboratory level (C. Cray, personal observation).[13] Significant interspecific differences including total white and blood cell counts and lymphocyte counts were reported in deer mice bred for use in laboratory studies.[14]

Sex

A significantly lower packed cell volume and red blood cell count were reported in captive female bald eagles.[5] In a multiyear study of burrowing parrots, male birds were reported to have higher heterophil/lymphocyte ratios.[15] Males were also reported to have better body condition. In a recent study of horned guan,[16] juvenile males were found to have higher red blood cell parameters. This finding was also observed in 2 species of endangered parrots from Brazil (red-capped parrot and the vinaceous Amazon parrot).[9] In the latter study, females were also reported to have a higher number of lymphocytes. In contrast, in a large study of mute swans,[8] no hematologic differences were reported between males and females. In a study of Galapagos penguins,[17] samples from males were found to have a higher packed cell volume and females had 2-fold higher eosinophil counts. No sex differences were reported for packed cell volume in Chinese 3-striped box turtles but higher red blood cell parameters were observed in male yellow-marginated box turtles.[11,18] Higher eosinophil counts were also observed in males in the latter study. In a study of aged Siberian hamsters,[19] no hematologic differences by sex were observed.

Location/husbandry

A recent study of horned guan under human care from 3 facilities reported differences related to husbandry, although they were found to be small and not clinically significant.[16] Broad RI were generated for outbred and inbred strains of albino mice from several different vendors, but the investigators acknowledged a variability among white blood cell parameters by institution.[20] Significant differences in white blood and red blood cell parameters were observed in Wistar rats obtained from 2 different breeders.[21] In wildlife studies, differences are often reported when comparing results from wild and captive animals. Higher neutrophil counts were reported in wild-caught versus aquarium-housed sturgeon.[22]

Circadian and seasonal variability

Seasonal changes have been reported in clinical chemistry parameters in avian species (especially related to egg laying).[12,23] In a multiyear study of burrowing parrots, a long dry season dictated by La Niña resulted in a high heterophil/lymphocyte ratio.[15] This finding continued to be present until the start of warm rainy seasons a few years later. Molting and egg laying have been shown to affect hematologic values in many avian species, including kestrels and penguins.[24,25] Packed cell volume and heterophil/lymphocyte counts were found to vary with season in captive Spix macaws.[26] Marked seasonal related changes in red blood cell parameters and monocytes were reported in the yellow-marginated box turtle.[18]

Preanalytical Procedures

The control of preanalytical conditions is key to producing RI that are based on as small variation as possible. The conditions in which samples are acquired should be part of a formal procedure, and deviations should be noted in case data from some samples may represent outliers. At minimum, the following items should be part of this preplanning stage.[27]

Patient preparation and handling
Although fasting samples are not commonly obtained in avian and exotic species, differences in handling can be considered a major factor. The induction of a stress hemogram is well described in the avian literature.[28,29]

Sample collection
This item is related to site of collection, sample type, storage, and period for analysis. Extended RI for ferrets were recently generated on a large sample set.[30] The investigators reported significant differences versus other literature that were, in part, attributed to blood sampling methods. Ethylenediaminetetraacetic acid (EDTA) and heparin are commonly and often interchangeably used in preparing avian hematology samples but have known differences.[31] These anticoagulants as well as sodium citrate have been examined in blood samples from macaws and pythons.[32] With delays in smear preparation and manual counting (by smear and by the Natt and Herrick method), the investigators reported that avian samples should be analyzed within 12 hours and reptile samples should be analyzed within 24 hours. Storage was recommended at 4°C. These types of parameters have also been examined in small mammals. Blood samples from rats and mice that were collected in EDTA were found to be stable regardless of storage temperature (refrigeration and ambient temperature) for 48 hours.[33] This finding was inclusive of automated analysis, including white and red blood cell counts, hemoglobin, and hematocrit. In another study, although a similar stability was reported for automated analysis components, significant changes were observed in blood smears that were prepared 24 hours or later. The investigators recommended that complete blood counts be conducted within 6 hours. If hematologic analysis occurs in-clinic, these recommendations can likely be adhered to. However, hematologic analyses are often performed at the reference laboratory level with a minimum 24-hour delay. Thus, laboratory-derived RI should reflect the type of samples that are most commonly analyzed (ie, anticoagulant, time before analysis, storage).

Analytical error
Although samples are obtained and analyzed for RI generation, additional records, including coefficient of variation analysis, should be conducted. It is important that the quality of analysis is continuous throughout the RI project.

Analytical Procedures
As part of the description of RI demographics, the analytical procedures used to obtain the results should be well detailed. Manual hematologic methods are used for avian and reptile samples, inclusive of estimates and 2 types of total white blood cell counting methods. There are methodological differences between the Unopette/Leukopet system, which uses phloxine, and the Natt and Herrick system, which uses methyl violet.[31,34] All 3 require trained technical staff for best reproducibility, but manual methods lack precision. In addition, preanalytical error may result in skewed differential counts, which affects final total white blood cell calculations. Published intervals should clearly state the method that has been used. Transference and multicenter RI are difficult to obtain by these methods. Automated methods using the Cell-Dyn 3500 analyzer (Abbott Laboratories, Abbott Park, IL, USA) have been reported and implanted in some laboratories.[35] Although automation generally brings greater precision, only total granulocyte counts were observed to have a good level of precision. Given the lack of standard automated method, a recent investigation focused on the application of high-throughput image cytometry.[36] As this technology becomes more widely used in veterinary laboratories, additional studies should be completed to address the full application to avian and reptile hematology.

Small and exotic mammal hematology is more often completed using automated analyzers to provide, at minimum, total cell counts, hemoglobin, and hematocrit levels. Manual white blood cell counts are still commonly performed for some exotic species, in which the leukocyte differential may represent a challenge because of unique cells (eg, heterophil in rabbits). In all mammals, there is significant concern for the random error associated with manual assessments.[37] When automated analyzers can be used to produce RI for mammalian populations, these intervals would be understood to be analyzer specific, given physical differences of analyzer operation, reagents, and calibration.[38,39] Analyzer information should always be provided in RI documentation.

Statistical Analysis

Statistical analyses used in the definition of RI should be well defined for users or readers of published intervals. Newly issued guidelines should be followed, as discussed in the next section.

CURRENT GUIDELINES FOR REFERENCE INTERVAL GENERATION

The ASVCP issued strong guidelines for the generation of RI in 2011.[27] These guidelines were the culmination of a detailed review by the ASVCP Quality Assurance and Laboratory Standards Committee and evolving standards for RI generation in human clinical pathology. Population-based RI have always been favored in the literature and in practical use, with the first recommendation for RI methods issued after the impaneling of an expert committee by the International Federation of Clinical Chemistry (IFCC) in 1970.[40] Panel reviews of this subject occurred over the years, most recently by the Clinical and Laboratory Standards Institute (CLSI) in 2008.[41] These joint IFCC-CLSI guidelines have been adopted by the ASVCP and involve the recommendation, especially in veterinary medicine, that RI be generated a priori or in a prospective study, in which all influences on interval generation can be best controlled. These guidelines form the gold standard of analysis, although other methods of RI generation are potentially applicable to veterinary medicine (**Table 2**).

Table 2
Methods for RI generation

RI Methodology	Description
n≥120, nonparametric	Gold standard
n = 40–120, robust	Lower sample size results in bias, robust method can be used with Gaussian or non-Gaussian distribution
n = 40–120, parametric	Lower sample size results in bias, data need to have Gaussian distribution even if they require transformation
n = 20–40, robust	Lower sample size results in bias, 90% confidence interval should be calculated, minimum-maximum values should be shown
n = 10–20	List all data points, include histogram and mean/median
Transference and multicenter	Analytical methods and patient demographics need to be equivocal
Indirect estimation	Acknowledgment of results from clinically abnormal animals are present in the data set; large sample sizes are possible
Index of individuality	Subject-based rather than population-based RI

Outlier Identification

Histograms or box plots are common tools that can be used to help identify outliers in a large sample set. Finding outliers may highlight issues with data transcription, sample quality, and misidentified healthy animals within the reference population. Due diligence should be given to identify any issue with a possible outlier before inclusion in the final data set. During statistical analysis, the data set should have Gaussian distribution and be analyzed by tests such as Dixon-Reed or Tukey.[1] The ASVCP recommends that outliers should not be indiscriminately removed and that appropriate outlier tests should be conducted for the type of sample set that is being analyzed.[27]

Data Distribution

Data distribution is a key influence of outlier identification and in the choice of RI method. Several methods, including Kolmogorov-Smirnov and Anderson-Darling, can be used, and if the distribution is not Gaussian, the data can be transformed and reanalyzed.[27] In human laboratory medicine, in which data points can often be in excess, data distribution can also be examined after partitioning the data by age or gender as well as other demographics, such as race, ethnicity, and lifestyle.[42]

Nonparametric Methods

When a sample size meets the recommended level of greater than 120, nonparametric methods are recommended, regardless of data distribution. A full reference sample set of 120 should be the goal of any RI study. Increased imprecision has been reported with smaller sample sets.[1,43]

Robust Methods

When sample size is between 40 and 120, the robust method is recommended; it can be used with non-Gaussian data.[27] The robust method is often found on clinical laboratory software, including an Excel freeware.[44]

Parametric Methods

When a Gaussian distribution is present, the parametric method can be used for sample sets between 40 and 120.[27]

Limited Sample Size

Sample sets between 20 and 40 can be analyzed by the robust or parametric methods, but a histogram of the data should be included, as well as 90% confidence intervals for the upper and lower limits.[27] Samples sets obtained from fewer than 20 individuals should not be used for RI generation. A histogram and all values can be shown such that users can understand the likelihood of variation.

Transference, Multicenter Intervals, and Published Intervals

Transference involves the adoption of RI between laboratories that use comparable analytical methods and analyzers.[1,27] Users of this method must acknowledge that the reference population used to generate the RI was soundly investigated and the patient demographics between laboratories were also comparable. A method comparison study should be undertaken before adoption as well as a thorough pre-evaluation with healthy animals from the laboratory's clientele.[45] In human clinical laboratory medicine, an analysis of 20 reference individuals from the laboratory's own population is conducted.[42] If more than 2 of the 20 tested values fall outside the RI that is under examination, the RI cannot be transferred to the new laboratory.

Given the mostly manual methodology involved in avian and reptile hematology, this method does not have a strong foundation nor does the use of multicenter-derived RI from a coalition of laboratories. These methods have greater applicability in procedures, including clinical chemistry and automated hematology.

In avian, exotic, and wildlife medicine, the use of published RI is especially tenuous. Although there are many publications in this area, sample size is often low, and animal demographics are not well described. Recently, many journals have been moving forward in requiring at least partial adherence to the ASVCP guidelines and presentation.[46] Methods sections of such publications should be closely examined for all of the influences on RI described in the previous section.

Validation and Reassessment

Newly generated RI should always be subject to validation. By this method, the RI should be examined during analyses of test results from the laboratory's regular patient population. As part of the permanent record, patient demographics, sample types, and analytical methods should be documented.

Once RI are generated, it should be recognized that RI should always be periodically examined. Bovine hematology RI were the focus of a detailed study of data from 1957 to 2006.[38] With the purchase of a new hematology analyzer, the investigators identified significant RI differences, which may have been related to the reference populations, analyzer, or statistical methods. In an extended study, influences including a possible genetic shift, underlying diseases and infections, and husbandry practices were all considered in the changes found in intervals for complete blood count over a 50-year period.

ALTERNATIVE METHODS TO TRADITIONAL REFERENCE INTERVALS

Given the challenges in obtaining data from 120 unique samples for nonparametric RI generation, alternative methods in RI generation may be more viable when working with smaller sample sets or repeated measures in avian and exotic animals. These intervals, although not completely vetted, may provide, at minimum, temporary intervals until a proper RI threshold can be met.

A Posteriori Determination

RI studies are recommended to be conducted prospectively when there can be the most awareness regarding sample demographics, analytical errors, and so forth. However, if the key elements to RI generation can be derived from banked data, RI may be suitable for use.[1]

Indirect Determination

The indirect method has an appeal, because it makes use of large databases of data from animals with unknown health status.[1,47] This method is generally viewed with caution, because it goes against ASVCP guidelines that the reference population should be clearly defined and that care should be taken in sample acquisition and processing.[42] However, there have been several positive reports based on human and veterinary data.[47-51] The first step in this method is analyzing a sample set of data obtained from known clinically normal animals. Given the RI that are generated from this data set, lower and upper fences can be set on the large undefined dataset. Outliers are removed, and then, the data set is analyzed by the routine recommended methods.

Recently, this method was reported for use in the generation of hematology and clinical chemistry RI in several psittacine species.[52] Seven species were examined, with sample size varying from approximately 350 to 2300. Compared with clinical expectations and poorly defined published reference ranges, the RI appeared to represent a broader range for many hematology measures. Higher total white blood cell counts and heterophil counts were present, possibly reflecting the inclusion of birds with clinical or subclinical disease or birds with a stress response. This finding was noted especially in the white blood cell intervals generated for the macaw, which has previously been described to have increased counts with the stress of transport to the animal clinic.[28] Some biochemical results reflected more narrow ranges versus clinical expectations. Overall, the results indicate that the indirect method of RI generation should not be indiscriminately used, but perhaps, it could be used to provide some rough estimates for some species until adequate sample size and animal demographics can be reached for more accurate RI generation. Thus, the final evaluation of this method in avian species was not as positive as that reported in large populations of sheep.[47] Concerns with the avian database may have been more heavily represented by samples from clinically abnormal birds, because routine annual blood work is not common in avian and exotic animal medicine.

Index of Individuality

When repeated measures are available, another alternative method to the generation of RI is the calculation of the index of individuality. It has been reported that variations in traditional population-based RI are wider than that observed in single animals or humans.[53–55] In the index of individuality method, the variation in repeated measures is used in a calculation; if the result is less than 0.6, this indicates that there is a high degree of individuality for results for that analyte, and regular RI have limited applicability but subject-based RI has value. If the variation is found to be higher, then population-based RI should be used.[53]

Individual biological variation studies have been conducted in birds. Over a few months, biochemical parameters were repeatedly measured in racing pigeons, but only total protein met the standards set by the index of individuality calculation.[56] An extended study[57] was also conducted in budgerigars, but the data indicated that population-based RI would be preferable. Repeated measures inclusive of routine hematology and biochemistry for 41 eagles were obtained over a 12-year period.[5] A high degree of individuality was reported for all analytes, except for γ globulins (determined by plasma protein electrophoresis). Biological variation was also examined in Dumeril monitors.[58] Analysis of data for several biochemical analytes showed that population-based RI is ill advised for this species. Clinical chemistry parameters obtained from automated analyzers may be better suited to index of individuality calculations versus results obtained from manual hematology methods, which inherently have a higher variation in results.

SUMMARY

When properly formulated and implemented, RI can be "the most widely used medical decision-making tool."[59] Although veterinary medicine has lagged behind human clinical laboratory medicine in RI guidelines, recent advances by the ASVCP have provided a good framework for RI generation, including in those species with limited sample size. Alternative methods to RI generation also can have application to avian and exotic species. Regardless of the method selected, patient demographics, preanalytical standards, and analytical methods should be well documented to understand potential RI bias and to provide the best chance for the adoption of RI by laboratories and clinicians.

REFERENCES

1. Geffre A, Friedrichs K, Harr K, et al. Reference values: a review. Vet Clin Pathol 2009;38(3):288–98. http://dx.doi.org/10.1111/j.1939-165X.2009.00179.x.
2. Clubb SL, Schubot RM, Joyner K. Hematologic and serum biochemical reference intervals in juvenile eclectus parrots. Journal of Avian Medicine & Surgery 1991;4:218–25.
3. Clubb SL, Schubot RM, Joyner K. Hematologic and serum biochemical reference intervals in juvenile macaws. Journal of Avian Medicine & Surgery 1991;5:154–62.
4. Clubb SL, Shubot RM, Joyner K. Hematologic and serum biochemical reference intervals in juvenile cockatoos. Journal of Avian Medicine & Surgery 1991;5:16–26.
5. Jones MP, Arheart KL, Cray C. Reference intervals, longitudinal analyses, and index of individuality of commonly measured laboratory variables in captive bald eagles (*Haliaeetus leucocephalus*). J Avian Med Surg 2014; 28(2):118–26.
6. Dujowich M, Mazet JK, Zuba JR. Hematologic and biochemical reference ranges for captive California condors (*Gymnogyps californianus*). J Zoo Wildl Med 2005;36(4):590–7.
7. Hawkey C, Hart MG, Samour HJ. Age-related haematological changes and haemopathological responses in Chilean flamingos (*Phoenicopterus chiliensis*). Avian Pathol 1984;13(2):223–9. pii:784689311.
8. Dolka B, Wlodarczyk R, Zbikowski A, et al. Hematological parameters in relation to age, sex and biochemical values for mute swans (*Cygnus olor*). Vet Res Commun 2014;38(2):93–100. http://dx.doi.org/10.1007/s11259-014-9589-y.
9. Schmidt EM, Lange RR, Ribas JM, et al. Hematology of the red-capped parrot (*Pionopsitta pileata*) and vinaceous Amazon parrot (*Amazona vinacea*) in captivity. J Zoo Wildl Med 2009;40(1):15–7.
10. Rousselet E, Stacy NI, LaVictoire K, et al. Hematology and plasma biochemistry analytes in five age groups of immature, captive-reared loggerhead sea turtles (*Caretta caretta*). J Zoo Wildl Med 2013;44(4):859–74.
11. Grioni A, Ho KK, Karraker NE, et al. Blood clinical biochemistry and packed cell volume of the Chinese three-striped box turtle, *Cuora trifasciata* (Reptilia: Geoemydidae). J Zoo Wildl Med 2014;45(2):228–38.
12. Scope A, Frommlet F, Schwendenwein I. Circadian and seasonal variability and influence of sex and race on eight clinical chemistry parameters in budgerigars (*Melopsittacus undulatus*, Shaw 1805). Res Vet Sci 2005;78(1):85–91. http://dx.doi.org/10.1016/j.rvsc.2004.07.001.
13. Polo FJ, Peinado VI, Viscor G, et al. Hematologic and plasma chemistry values in captive psittacine birds. Avian Dis 1998;42(3):523–35.
14. Wiedmeyer CE, Crossland JP, Veres M, et al. Hematologic and serum biochemical values of 4 species of *Peromyscus* mice and their hybrids. J Am Assoc Lab Anim Sci 2014;53(4):336–43.
15. Plischke A, Quillfeldt P, Lubjuhn T, et al. Leucocytes in adult burrowing parrots *Cyanoliseus patagonus* in the wild: variation between contrasting breeding seasons, gender, and individual condition. J Ornithol 2010;151:347–54.
16. Cornejo J, Richardson D, Perez JG, et al. Hematologic and plasma biochemical reference values of the horned guan, *Oreophasis derbianus*. J Zoo Wildl Med 2014;45(1):15–22.

17. Travis EK, Vargas FH, Merkel J, et al. Hematology, serum chemistry, and serology of Galapagos penguins (*Spheniscus mendiculus*) in the Galapagos islands, Ecuador. J Wildl Dis 2006;42(3):625–32. pii:42/3/625.

18. Yang PY, Yu PH, Wu SH, et al. Seasonal hematology and plasma biochemistry reference range values of the yellow-marginated box turtle (*Cuora flavomarginata*). J Zoo Wildl Med 2014;45(2):278–86.

19. McKeon GP, Nagamine CM, Ruby NF, et al. Hematologic, serologic, and histologic profile of aged Siberian hamsters (*Phodopus sungorus*). J Am Assoc Lab Anim Sci 2011;50(3):308–16.

20. Serfilippi LM, Pallman DR, Russell B. Serum clinical chemistry and hematology reference values in outbred stocks of albino mice from three commonly used vendors and two inbred strains of albino mice. Contemp Top Lab Anim Sci 2003;42(3):46–52.

21. Kampfmann I, Bauer N, Johannes S, et al. Differences in hematologic variables in rats of the same strain but different origin. Vet Clin Pathol 2012;41(2):228–34. http://dx.doi.org/10.1111/j.1939-165X.2012.00427.x.

22. DiVincenti L Jr, Priest H, Walker KJ, et al. Comparison of select hematology and serum chemistry analytes between wild-caught and aquarium-housed lake sturgeon (*Acipenser fulvescens*). J Zoo Wildl Med 2013;44(4):957–64.

23. de Carvalho FM, Gaunt SD, Kearney MT, et al. Reference intervals of plasma calcium, phosphorus, and magnesium for African grey parrots (*Psittacus erithacus*) and Hispaniolan parrots (*Amazona ventralis*). J Zoo Wildl Med 2009;40(4):675–9.

24. Mazzaro LM, Meegan J, Sarran D, et al. Molt-associated changes in hematologic and plasma biochemical values and stress hormone levels in African penguins (*Spheniscus demersus*). J Avian Med Surg 2013;27(4):285–93.

25. Rehder NB, Bird DM. Annual profiles of blood packed cell volumes of captive American kestrels. Can J Zool 1983;61:2550–5.

26. Foldenauer U, Borjal RJ, Deb A, et al. Hematologic and plasma biochemical values of Spix's macaws (*Cyanopsitta spixii*). J Avian Med Surg 2007;21(4):275–82.

27. Friedrichs K, Barnhart K, Blanco J, et al. Guidelines for the determination of reference intervals (RI) in veterinary species. Available at: http://www.asvcp.org/pubs/pdf/RI%20Guidelines%20For%20ASVCP%20website.pdf. Accessed August 8, 2014.

28. Speer BL, Kass PH. The influence of travel of hematologic parameters in hyacinth macaws. Proc Annu Conf Assoc Avian Vet. 1995. p. 43–9.

29. Parga ML, Pendl H, Forbes NA. The effect of transport on hematologic parameters in trained and untrained Harris's hawks (*Parabuteo unicinctus*) and peregrine falcons (*Falco peregrinus*). J Avian Med Surg 2001;15(3):162–9.

30. Hein J, Spreyer F, Sauter-Louis C, et al. Reference ranges for laboratory parameters in ferrets. Vet Rec 2012;171(9):218. http://dx.doi.org/10.1136/vr.100628.

31. Walberg J. White blood cell counting techniques in birds. Journal of Exotic Pet Medicine 2001;10(2):72–6.

32. Harr KE, Raskin RE, Heard DJ. Temporal effects of 3 commonly used anticoagulants on hematologic and biochemical variables in blood samples from macaws and Burmese pythons. Vet Clin Pathol 2005;34(4):383–8.

33. O'Donnoghue JM, Strong MA, Detolla LJ. Effects of varying storage time and temperature on stability of complete blood count measurements. Contemp Top Lab Anim Sci 1998;57(6):52–60.

34. Dein JF, Wilson A, Fischer D, et al. Avian leukocyte counting using the hemocytometer. J Zoo Wildl Med 1994;25(3):423–37.

35. Lilliehook I, Wall H, Tauson R, et al. Differential leukocyte counts determined in chicken blood using the Cell-Dyn 3500. Vet Clin Pathol 2004; 33(3):133–8.
36. Beaufrere H, Ammersbach M, Tully TN Jr. Complete blood cell count in psittaciformes by using high-throughput image cytometry: a pilot study. J Avian Med Surg 2013;27(3):211–7.
37. Kjelgaard-Hansen M, Jensen AL. Is the inherent imprecision of manual leukocyte differential counts acceptable for quantitative purposes? Vet Clin Pathol 2006;35(3):268–70.
38. George JW, Snipes J, Lane VM. Comparison of bovine hematology reference intervals from 1957 to 2006. Vet Clin Pathol 2010;39(2):138–48. http://dx.doi. org/10.1111/j.1939-165X.2009.00208.x.
39. Weingand KW, Odioso LW, Dameron GW, et al. Hematology analyzer comparison: Ortho ELT-8/ds vs. Baker 9000 for healthy dogs, mice, and rats. Vet Clin Pathol 1992;21(1):10–4.
40. Solberg HE, Grasbeck R. Reference values. Adv Clin Chem 1989;27:1–79.
41. Horowitz GL, Altaie S, Boyd JC, et al. 3rd edition. Defining, establishing, and verifying reference intervals in the clinical laboratory; approved guidelines, vol. 28. Wayne (PA): Clinical and Laboratory Standards Institute; 2008. no. 3.
42. Ceriotti F. Prerequisites for use of common reference intervals. Clin Biochem Rev 2007;28(3):115–21.
43. Geffre A, Braun JP, Trumel C, et al. Estimation of reference intervals from small samples: an example using canine plasma creatinine. Vet Clin Pathol 2009; 38(4):477–84. http://dx.doi.org/10.1111/j.1939-165X.2009.00155.x.
44. Geffre A, Concordet D, Braun JP, et al. Reference value advisor: a new freeware set of macroinstructions to calculate reference intervals with Microsoft Excel. Vet Clin Pathol 2011;40(1):107–12. http://dx.doi.org/10.1111/j.1939-165X.2011. 00287.x.
45. Jensen AL, Kjelgaard-Hansen M. Method comparison in the clinical laboratory. Vet Clin Pathol 2006;35(3):276–86.
46. Cray C. Reference intervals: new guidelines for an essential resource. Vet Rec 2012;171(9):215–6. http://dx.doi.org/10.1136/vr.e5811.
47. Dimauro C, Bonelli P, Nicolussi P, et al. Estimating clinical chemistry reference values based on an existing data set of unselected animals. Vet J 2008; 178(2):278–81. http://dx.doi.org/10.1016/j.tvjl.2007.08.002.
48. Ilcol YO, Aslan D. Use of total patient data for indirect estimation of reference intervals for 40 clinical chemical analytes in turkey. Clin Chem Lab Med 2006; 44(7):867–76. http://dx.doi.org/10.1515/CCLM.2006.139.
49. Horn PS, Feng L, Li Y, et al. Effect of outliers and nonhealthy individuals on reference interval estimation. Clin Chem 2001;47(12):2137–45.
50. Ferre-Masferrer M, Fuentes-Arderiu X, Puchal-Ane R. Indirect reference limits estimated from patients' results by three mathematical procedures. Clin Chim Acta 1999;279(1–2):97–105.
51. Concordet D, Geffre A, Braun JP, et al. A new approach for the determination of reference intervals from hospital-based data. Clin Chim Acta 2009;405(1–2): 43–8. http://dx.doi.org/10.1016/j.cca.2009.03.057.
52. Tang F, Messinger S, Cray C. Use of an indirect sampling method to produce reference intervals for hematologic and biochemical analyses in psittaciform species. J Avian Med Surg 2013;27(3):194–203.
53. Harris EK. Effects of intra- and interindividual variation on the appropriate use of normal ranges. Clin Chem 1974;20(12):1535–42.

54. Walton RM. Subject-based reference values: biological variation, individuality, and reference change values. Vet Clin Pathol 2012;41(2):175–81.
55. Costongs GM, Janson PC, Bas BM, et al. Short-term and long-term intra-individual variations and critical differences of clinical chemical laboratory parameters. J Clin Chem Clin Biochem 1985;23(1):7–16.
56. Scope A, Schwendenwein I, Gabler C. Short-term variations of biochemical parameters in racing pigeons (*Columba livia*). J Avian Med Surg 2002;16(1):10–5.
57. Scope A, Schwendenwein I, Frommlet F. Biological variation, individuality and critical differences in eight biochemical blood constituents in budgerigars (*Melopsittacus undulatus*). Vet Rec 2006;159:839–43.
58. Bertelsen MF, Kjelgaard-Hansen M, Howell JR, et al. Short-term biological variation of clinical chemical values in Dumeril's monitors (*Varanus dumerili*). J Zoo Wildl Med 2007;38(2):217–21.
59. Horn PS, Pesce AJ. Reference intervals: an update. Clin Chim Acta 2003; 334:5–23.

Evaluation of the Blood Film

Terry W. Campbell, MS, DVM, PhD

KEYWORDS

- Blood • Cells • Hematology • Mammal • Bird • Reptile • Amphibian • Fish

KEY POINTS

- A single drop of blood can provide valuable information in the assessment of the exotic animal patient by the examination of a properly prepared blood film.
- A blood film will reveal important erythrocyte abnormalities, such as changes in cell shape and color, presence of inclusions, and, in the case of lower vertebrates, changes in the position of the cell nucleus.
- A differential leukocyte count and detection of white blood cell abnormalities can be obtained from a stained blood film.
- Thrombocyte numbers and morphology are discerned from properly prepared blood films, in addition to mammalian platelets.
- A blood film can also reveal the presence of blood parasites and other infectious agents.

Evaluation of cell morphology in the stained blood film is an important part of hematology and the evaluation of the exotic animal patient. Often, the stained blood film is the only component of hematology available to the exotic animal veterinarian because of a small sample size. A single drop of blood can provide valuable information in the assessment of the patient.

A properly prepared blood film should not extend to the edges of the slide and will have a thick body that tapers into a feathered edge (**Fig. 1**). The best cell morphology lies just behind the feathered edge in the monolayer area. It is difficult to examine cells in the thick part of the blood film because they superimpose on each other, and the leukocytes appear rounded and not able to expand and flatten out (making them all resemble lymphocytes). Examination of cells in the feathered-edge area will reveal artifacts such as ruptured cells and, in the case of mammalian blood films, lack of erythrocyte central pallor.

A blood film made from a drop of non-anticoagulated blood placed on a slide immediately after collection is preferred over a blood sample exposed to an anticoagulant.

Department of Clinical Sciences, College of Veterinary Medicine and Biomedical Sciences, Colorado State University, 300 West Drake Road, Fort Collins, CO 80523, USA
E-mail address: Terry.Campbell@colostate.edu

Vet Clin Exot Anim 18 (2015) 117–135
http://dx.doi.org/10.1016/j.cvex.2014.09.001

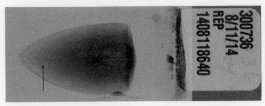

Fig. 1. Blood film with a thick body tapering to a feathered edge from a lizard (*Pogona vitticeps*) stained with Wright-Giemsa stain. The best cell morphology lies just behind the feathered edge in the monolayer area (*arrow*).

Anticoagulants, such as heparin and citrate, may affect the staining quality of the blood film. The anticoagulant EDTA (ethylenediaminetetraacetic acid) may cause hemolysis or cause the blood to clot in some species, such as birds in the crow family (corvids) or cartilaginous fish (elasmobranchs), rendering the sample useless. Once the film has been prepared, it should be dried immediately. In most settings, this is accomplished by waving the slide in the air; however, in high humidity the use of a commercially available slide warmer or a hair dryer set on a low (warm) setting held in front of the slide may be needed to properly dry the slide to prevent drying artifacts, such as excessive crenation of the red blood cells. Blood slides should be labeled with the animal identification information and the date. Romanowsky stains, such as Wright or Wright-Giemsa, are commonly used for the evaluation of hemic cytology.

At low magnification (using a 10× or 20× objective), an experienced cytologist can subjectively estimate the leukocyte concentration on a blood film as being low (leukopenia), normal, or high (leukocytosis) before examination of the cells using the 100× (oil-immersion) objective (**Fig. 2**). Several formulas for estimating the total leukocyte and thrombocyte concentrations from a blood film have been proposed; however, none are accurate or precise and should not be used in reporting leukocyte and thrombocyte numbers. The morphology of the 3 major cell types (erythrocytes, leukocytes, and platelets or thrombocytes) is best evaluated at higher magnifications.

A differential leukocyte count is obtained by counting a minimum of 100 consecutively encountered white blood cells in the monolayer area of the blood film. For most species, the cells are classified as neutrophils or heterophils (depending on species), eosinophils, basophils, lymphocytes, and monocytes, to obtain a relative percentage for each leukocyte type. Cells not readily identified can be placed into a sixth category of "other." Abnormalities in leukocyte morphologies are noted.

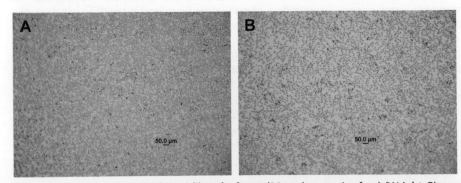

Fig. 2. (*A*) Leukocytosis in the blood film of a ferret (*Mustela putorius furo*) (Wright-Giemsa stain). (*B*) Leukocytosis in the blood film of a turtle (*Graptemys versa*) (Wright-Giemsa stain).

Evaluation of erythrocyte morphology is also made using high magnification. Important erythrocyte abnormalities include changes in cell shape, color changes, presence of inclusions, and, in the case of lower vertebrates, changes in the position of the cell nucleus.

Thrombocytes and mammalian platelets are evaluated under high magnification. Their numbers can be estimated as being adequate, low (thrombocytopenia), or high (thrombocytosis). In mammalian blood films, an average of 8 to 12 platelets per oil-immersion monolayer field is considered to be adequate. In lower vertebrates, such as birds and reptiles, an average of 1 to 2 thrombocytes per oil-immersion monolayer field is considered to be adequate, as these cells are larger than mammalian platelets. Lower numbers may indicate a true thrombocytopenia or excessive platelet clumping; the latter of which can be identified in the feathered-edge portion of the blood film. Evaluation of platelet morphology is made with special attention to size.

ERYTHROCYTES

Romanowsky-stained erythrocytes in mammalian blood films are anucleated, round (except those from camelids), biconcave discs that stain pink and often have a central area of pallor. As mammalian erythrocytes develop, there is an increase in hemoglobin synthesis, and during the final stages of maturation the nucleus undergoes degeneration and is extruded from the cells along with the organelles involved in metabolism. Reticulocytes are young erythrocytes in their final stage of maturation that have lost the nucleus, but have yet to lose ribosomes and mitochondria. When stained with new methylene blue or brilliant cresyl blue, these residual organelles aggregate into clumps of granular material referred to as reticulum, thus giving the cell the name reticulocyte. Reticulocytes in Wright-stained blood films appear blue and are called polychromatic cells.

Polychromatic cells in mammalian blood films are larger than mature erythrocytes and have a blue to reddish-blue cytoplasm. These cells may lack the classic discoid shape of mature red blood cell and have membranous folds.

The mean erythrocyte diameter of many small mammals ranges between 5 and 7 μm. The erythrocytes of small mammals, such as true rodents (ie, rats, *Rattus norvegicus*; mice, *Mus musculus*; gerbils, *Meriones unguiculatus*; and hamsters, *Mesocricetus auratus*) have a relatively short half-life (45–68 days) compared with larger mammals, such as dogs (100–115 days) and cats (73 days); as a result, their blood comparatively has a higher concentration of reticulocytes, so the presence of a greater degree of polychromasia and anisocytosis on the blood film is expected.[1–3] In general, 1% to 5% reticulocytes are expected in adult nonanemic rodents. On the opposite end of the spectrum, horses (with an erythrocyte life span of 140–145 days) do not release reticulocytes.

Diagnostically, the important morphologic characteristics of mammalian erythrocytes include polychromatic, hypochromic, microcytic, and macrocytic erythrocytes; poikilocytosis; and red blood cell inclusions. Knowing the packed cell volume is important in the detection of anemia, and evaluation of the blood film will aid in the determination of a regenerative or nonregenerative anemia. Polychromatic erythrocytes (reticulocytes) are young erythrocytes that have been released into circulation early, and therefore are larger and more basophilic in color compared with mature erythrocytes (**Fig. 3**). The degree of polychromasia (total number of polychromatic erythrocytes) will aid in the determination of the cause of an anemia. For example, an increase in polychromatic erythrocytes occurs with blood loss and blood-destruction anemias, whereas a decrease or lack of polychromasia is observed in anemias caused by erythroid hypoplasia or in an aplastic anemia.

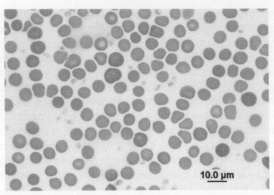

Fig. 3. Polychromatic erythrocytes (*blue-staining cells*) in the blood film of a domestic rat (*Rattus norvegicus*) (Wright-Giemsa stain).

Hypochromasia in the mammalian blood film is indicated by pale-staining erythrocytes with an increased area of central pallor. Hypochromatic erythrocytes indicate a state of iron deficiency. Iron deficiency in adult mammals is generally the result of chronic blood loss caused by bloodsucking parasites, gastrointestinal ulcers, inflammatory bowel disease, or neoplasms. Iron-deficiency anemia in very young mammals is due to inadequate dietary iron.

Electronic methods are better at determining the size of erythrocytes than are human eyes; however, when one has only a blood film to evaluate, the presence of large (macrocytic) and small (microcytic) red blood cells or anisocytosis may be apparent. Microcytic erythrocytes occur most commonly with iron-deficiency anemia or in iron-metabolism disorders. The most common cause of an increased number of macrocytic erythrocytes is an increase in polychromatic erythrocytes.

Poikilocytosis refers to an increased number of abnormally shaped erythrocytes. The important changes in the shape of mammalian erythrocytes include spiculated red blood cells and spherocytes. Fragmented red blood cells or schistocytes are spiculated cells caused by shearing forces during intravascular trauma, such as those caused by fibrin strands formed with disseminated intravascular coagulopathy or hemangiosarcoma, or from oxidative damage from iron-deficiency anemia. Keratocytes are iron-deficient red blood cells with 2 or more spicules that form during oxidative injury. Schistocytes form when the spicules fragment from the keratocytes.

Acanthocytes are spiculated mammalian erythrocytes that result from lipid metabolism changes in the cell membrane. Acanthocytes (also known as spur cells) possess unevenly distributed irregular spicules of variable lengths and diameters. Echinocytes or burr cells resemble acanthocytes, but have numerous short, evenly spaced spicules that are uniform in size and shape. Echinocytes are often artifacts and are a sign of crenation (a result of slow drying of blood films); however, they may also be seen with pathologic conditions such as renal disease, lymphoma, and rattlesnake envenomation.

Spherocytes appear as small, dark-staining erythrocytes that lack a central pallor. Spherocytes are more easily detected in species such as members of the family Canidae that have larger erythrocytes and prominent central pallor. Spherocytes are suggestive of immune-mediated hemolytic anemia.

Important structures in or on mammalian erythrocytes include Heinz bodies, basophilic stippling, nucleated erythrocytes, and Howell-Jolly bodies. Heinz bodies are small, eccentric, single to multiple pale structures that often protrude slightly from the red cell margins. Heinz bodies are caused by oxidative denaturation of hemoglobin, and can be associated with certain plant chemicals (onions and garlic), drugs (acetaminophen and propofol), and diseases such as lymphoma and hyperthyroidism. Basophilic stippling appears in the erythrocyte as small basophilic granules within the cytoplasm of the cell.

Basophilic stippling is commonly associated with erythrocyte regeneration, and is commonly found in blood films from healthy mammals such as gerbils. Basophilic stippling may also be associated with nonanemic animals with lead poisoning, but this is generally a rare finding.

Nucleated erythrocytes are immature red blood cells sometimes found in mammalian blood films (**Fig. 4**). These cells are released at an early stage of maturation from the bone marrow, usually as part of a regenerative response to anemia or hypoxia. An inappropriate release of nucleated erythrocytes may be seen with lead poisoning or a myelodysplastic condition.

Howell-Jolly bodies are small, variably sized, round, dark-blue inclusions present in the cytoplasm of the erythrocyte (**Fig. 5**). These inclusions represent nuclear remnants that occur as part of a regenerative response, or may indicate suppressed splenic function. Howell-Jolly bodies are found in low numbers of red cells in the blood films of normal mice and rats.

Other abnormalities such as Rouleaux formation and red blood cell agglutination should also be reported. Rouleaux formation appears as linear stacking of erythrocytes, and is often associated with increased plasma proteins, such as immunoglobulins, in domestic mammals. Rouleaux formation is uncommon in some mammals, such as rats and mice, with inflammatory disease. Erythrocyte agglutination may be identified by the irregular to circular clumping of erythrocytes, and is associated with immune-mediated hemolytic anemia.

Erythrocytes of lower vertebrates, such as birds, reptiles, amphibians, and fish, should be evaluated based on size, shape, color, nuclear morphology, and position, in addition to the presence of cellular inclusions. In general, the mature erythrocytes of these animals are elliptical and have an elliptical, centrally positioned nucleus. The immature erythrocytes begin as nucleated spheres that turn into flattened ellipsoids during the final stages of maturation. Unlike mammalian erythrocytes, erythrocytes of lower vertebrates retain their nuclei where the nuclear chromatin is uniformly clumped, and becomes increasingly condensed with age. In Wright-stained

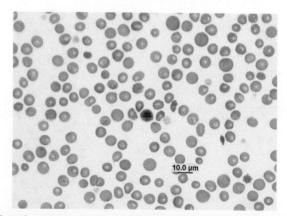

10.0 µm

Fig. 4. Nucleated erythrocyte in the blood film of an African hedgehog (*Atelerix albiventris*) (Wright-Giemsa stain).

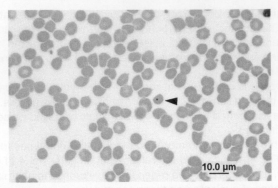

Fig. 5. A Howell-Jolly body (*arrowhead*) in the blood film of a ferret (*Mustela putorius furo*) (Wright-Giemsa stain).

blood films the nucleus stains purple, whereas the cytoplasm stains orange-pink with a uniform texture (**Fig. 6**).

Knowledge of avian hemic cytology in the blood film can serve as a model for evaluating the blood film from other lower vertebrate species. In most species of birds, erythrocyte shape is relatively uniform; however, the shape of the red blood cells from other lower vertebrates may be somewhat variable. Erythrocytes of reptiles are blunt-ended ellipsoidal cells with permanent, centrally positioned, oval to round nuclei containing dense purple chromatin. The erythrocytes of amphibians are large compared with those of other vertebrates, with sizes that vary from 10 to 70 μm in diameter. Most amphibian erythrocytes are nucleated and elliptical in shape, have a distinct nuclear bulge, and often have irregular nuclear margins. The erythrocytes of teleost fishes are similar in appearance to those of birds and reptiles (**Fig. 7**). The mature erythrocytes of elasmobranch fishes are also similar in appearance to avian and reptilian erythrocytes, but are much larger. Mature erythrocytes of some fish are biconvex with a central swelling that corresponds to the position of the nucleus, whereas other species have flattened biconcave erythrocytes.[4] The nuclei of fish erythrocytes can be large, and may occupy as much as one-fourth the cell volume or greater. The long axis of the nucleus is parallel to the long axis of the cell, except in a few species of fish that have round erythrocyte nuclei.

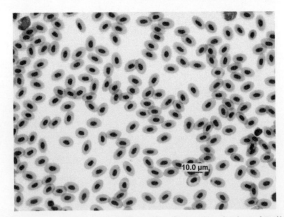

Fig. 6. Normal erythrocytes in the blood film of a domestic chicken (*Gallus gallus domesticus*) (Wright-Giemsa stain).

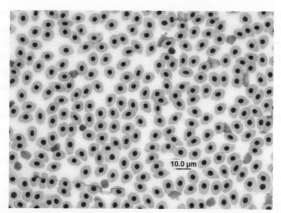

Fig. 7. Normal erythrocytes in the blood film of a fish (*Erimonax monachus*) (Wright-Giemsa stain).

Atypical erythrocytes may vary in both size and shape, and semiquantitative estimates of these changes can be made from evaluation of monolayer areas of the blood film (**Table 1**). The presence of macrocytes or microcytes should be noted during assessment of the blood film. The degree of variation in the size of erythrocytes (anisocytosis) can be scored from 1+ to 4+, based on the number of variably sized erythrocytes in a monolayer field (see **Table 1**).[5] Erythrocyte subpopulations have been reported in some species of birds (eg, ducks), in which larger erythrocytes most likely represent those most recently released from the hematopoietic tissue and smaller cells most likely represent the older, aging cells.[6] A slight variation in the size of erythrocytes (1+ anisocytosis) is considered normal for birds. A greater degree of anisocytosis, however, usually is observed in birds with a regenerative anemia, and is associated with polychromasia. Microcytic, hypochromic, nonregenerative anemia is often associated with chronic inflammatory diseases in birds, especially those with an infectious etiology.[7]

Minor deviations from the normal shape of avian erythrocytes (1+ poikilocytosis) are considered to be normal in the peripheral blood of birds, but marked poikilocytosis may indicate erythrocytic dysgenesis. For example, round erythrocytes with oval nuclei occasionally are found in the blood films of anemic birds and suggest a dysmaturation of the cell cytoplasm and nucleus, which may be a result of accelerated erythropoiesis.

Table 1
Semiquantitative microscopic evaluation of avian erythrocyte morphology[a]

	1+	2+	3+	4+
Anisocytosis	5–10	11–20	21–30	>30
Polychromasia	2–10	11–14	15–30	>30
Hypochromasia	1–2	3–5	6–10	>10
Poikilocytosis	5–10	11–20	21–50	>50
Erythroplastids	1–2	3–5	6–10	>10

[a] Based on the average number of abnormal cells per 1000× monolayer field.
Data from Campbell TW, Ellis CK. Avian and exotic animal hematology and cytology. 3rd edition. Ames (IA): Blackwell Publishing Ltd; 2007.

Variations in erythrocyte color include polychromasia and hypochromasia. Polychromatophilic erythrocytes are similar in size to mature erythrocytes and appear as reticulocytes when stained with vital stains, such as new methylene blue. The cytoplasm appears weakly basophilic, and the nucleus is less condensed than the nucleus of mature erythrocytes (**Fig. 8**). Polychromatophilic erythrocytes occur in low numbers (usually <5% of erythrocytes) in the peripheral blood of most normal birds. The degree of polychromasia can be graded according to the guideline presented in **Table 1**. Hypochromatic erythrocytes are abnormally pale in color compared with mature erythrocytes, and have an area of cytoplasmic pallor that is greater than half the cytoplasmic volume. These erythrocytes also may have cytoplasmic vacuoles and round, pyknotic nuclei. The degree of hypochromasia can be estimated using the scale presented in **Table 1**. The presence of many hypochromatic erythrocytes (ie, 2+ hypochromasia or greater) indicates an erythrocyte disorder such as iron deficiency.

The nucleus may vary in its location within the erythrocyte, and may contain indentions, protrusions, or constrictions. Micronuclei and nuclear budding are potential indices of environmental genotoxic exposure.[8,9] Chromophobic streaking suggestive of chromatolysis or achromic bands indicating nuclear fracture with displacement of the fragments may also be present.[10] Mitotic activity is occasionally noted in blood films, and is suggestive of a marked regenerative response or erythrocytic dyscrasia. Binucleate erythrocytes, when present in large numbers along with other features of red blood cell dyscrasia, are suggestive of neoplastic, viral, or genetic disease.[11] Anucleated erythrocytes (erythroplastids) or the presence of cytoplasmic fragments are occasionally noted in normal avian blood films.

LEUKOCYTES

The granulocytes of nondomestic mammals vary in appearance but can be classified as neutrophils or heterophils, eosinophils, and basophils.[12,13] Neutrophils contain cytoplasmic granules that stain neutral with Romanowsky stains, such as Wright or Wright-Giemsa stain. The 2 types of neutrophil commonly found in normal blood samples of most exotic mammal species are segmented neutrophils and small numbers of band neutrophils. Band neutrophils are immature neutrophils, and contain a smooth nucleus that has parallel sides and no constrictions in the nuclear membrane. Segmented neutrophils develop from band neutrophils. Neutrophils contain numerous

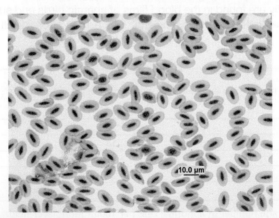

Fig. 8. Polychromasia (blue-staining erythrocytes) in the blood film of an eagle (*Aguila chrysaetos*) (Wright-Giemsa stain).

small granules that vary from colorless to pale-staining to dark-staining among different species of mammal. Neutrophils with a cytoplasm that typically stains diffusely pink with Romanowsky stains and contain variable numbers of larger eosinophilic granules are referred to as heterophils (**Fig. 9**). The granules of eosinophils become intensely eosinophilic with maturation as a result of the basic protein content with Wright or Wright-Giemsa staining. Mammalian basophils have characteristic cytoplasmic granules that are strongly basophilic in Romanowsky-stained blood films. In some species variation in the color of the granules occurs.

The avian heterophil is functionally equivalent to the mammalian neutrophil, and is the most abundant granulocyte of many species of birds. The nucleus (typically partially hidden by the cytoplasmic granules) of the mature heterophil is lobed (2–3 lobes), with coarse, clumped, purple-staining chromatin. The cytoplasm of normal mature heterophils appears colorless and contains granules that stain an eosinophilic color (dark orange to brown red) with Romanowsky stains (**Fig. 10**). Typically the cytoplasmic granules appear elongated (rod or spiculate shaped), but may also appear oval to round depending on the species.

Reptilian heterophils resemble those of birds, but are larger. These cells are typically round, with a colorless cytoplasm containing eosinophilic (bright orange), refractile, rod- to spindle-shaped cytoplasmic granules (**Fig. 11**). Occasionally degranulated heterophils can be found in the blood film of normal reptiles. The nucleus of the mature reptilian heterophil is typically eccentrically positioned in the cell, and is round to oval with densely clumped nuclear chromatin. However, some species of lizards have heterophils with lobed nuclei.

The nucleus of the avian eosinophil is lobed and usually stains darker than the nucleus of a heterophil, and the cytoplasm stains clear blue, in contrast to the colorless cytoplasm of normal mature heterophils (**Fig. 12**). The cytoplasmic granules are strongly eosinophilic in appearance and tend to stain more intensely in comparison with the granules of the heterophil on the same stained blood film. The granules are typically round in shape, although those of some avian species may be oval or elongated.

The eosinophils in most reptilian blood films are large round cells with light-blue cytoplasm, a round to oval (possibly lobed in some species of lizards), slightly eccentric nucleus, and large numbers of spherical eosinophilic cytoplasmic granules. The cytoplasmic granules of some reptilian species, such as *Iguana iguana*, stain blue with Romanowsky stains.

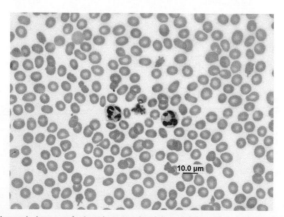

Fig. 9. Heterophils and clump of platelets in the blood film of a guinea pig (*Cavia porcellus*) (Wright-Giemsa stain).

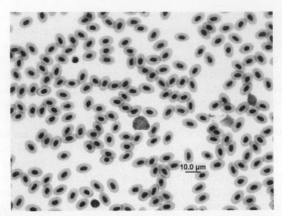

Fig. 10. Normal heterophil in the blood film of a domestic chicken (*Gallus gallus domesticus*) (Wright-Giemsa stain).

The basophils of birds and reptiles contain deeply metachromic granules that often obscure the nucleus. The nucleus is usually nonlobed, causing avian basophils to resemble mammalian mast cells (**Fig. 13**).

In general, amphibian granulocytes resemble those of mammals but are comparatively larger. Amphibian granulocytes are classified based on their appearance in blood smears stained with Wright-Giemsa and their resemblance to mammalian granulocytes; therefore, they have been classified as neutrophils, eosinophils, and basophils. Other classifications in the literature use heterophils instead of neutrophils.[12,14,15]

The term neutrophil has been frequently used to describe the predominant granulocyte of teleost fish, even if the granules in the cells do not stain neutral, because overall the cells resemble mammalian neutrophils when stained with Romanowsky stains. The cytoplasm of the mature piscine neutrophil is typically abundant and colorless, grayish, or slightly acidophilic in color, whereas the cytoplasm of immature neutrophils stains gray or blue-gray. Small granules may be present within the cytoplasm. Staining of the cytoplasmic granules is variable and depends on the species of fish or maturity

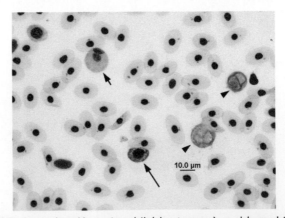

Fig. 11. Heterophils (*arrowheads*), eosinophil (*short arrow*), and basophil (*long arrow*) in the blood film of a turtle (*Trachemys scripta elegans*) (Wright-Giemsa stain).

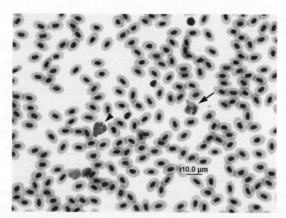

Fig. 12. An eosinophil (*arrow*) and normal heterophil (*arrowhead*) in the blood film of a domestic chicken (*Gallus gallus domesticus*) (Wright-Giemsa stain).

of the cell. The granules do not stain at all in most fish species, but may stain pale red, blue, or violet in others.[16] When present, eosinophils occur in low numbers that can be differentiated from neutrophils (or heterophils) by the presence of numerous round- to rod-shaped eosinophilic staining granules in a light-blue cytoplasm in films stained with Romanowsky stains. Basophils are rare in peripheral blood films of bony fish, and have been reported in only a few fish species.[17,18]

There is a considerable amount of confusion in the literature with regard to the naming of the various granulocytes found in the different species of elasmobranchs, partially because the granulocytes exhibit a marked variation in numbers and types between the species.[18–22] An attempt to standardize and simplify the nomenclature involving elasmobranch granulocytes has been offered using avian rather than mammalian terminology.[23] This system allows the granulocytes of elasmobranch fishes to be classified as heterophils, eosinophils, and basophils using the descriptive criteria for those cells in avian hematology. This scheme works well for some species; however, other elasmobranchs exhibit granulocytes that possess neutral-staining granules. These neutrophil-like granulocytes typically have an eccentric nonlobed

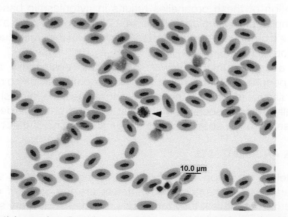

Fig. 13. A basophil (*arrowhead*) in the blood film of a hawk (*Buteo jamaicensis*) (Wright-Giemsa stain).

nucleus. It is not known whether these cells represent a fourth type of granulocyte or result from an artifact of the staining process.[23]

Monocytes are generally the largest leukocytes in peripheral blood films of animals, and do not vary grossly in appearance between species. The monocyte nucleus varies in shape (round or oval to lobed), and the moderately abundant cytoplasm is typically light blue-gray and may be vacuolated. The granules, when present, are very fine and appear azurophilic in Romanowsky-stained preparations.

The appearances of lymphocytes in the blood films of lower vertebrates resemble those of mammals. Their appearance may vary depending on the species, lymphocyte type, and degree of activation. Lymphocytes vary in size, color of cytoplasm (light to dark blue), and degree of nuclear chromatin condensation. Variability depends on the degree of antigenic stimulation and type of lymphocyte. The size of lymphocytes ranges from the size of an erythrocyte to the size a neutrophil or heterophil. The small lymphocytes are considered to be the inactive forms. Reactive lymphocytes have a slightly more abundant cytoplasm that stains basophilic, and nuclei that have clefts or are irregular in shape. These cells are considered to be B cells involved in immuno-globulin production.[24] Large lymphocytes that have an increased amount of light-blue cytoplasm and azurophilic granules that vary in size are considered to be T cells or natural killer cells.[25]

ACQUIRED CHANGES IN LEUKOCYTE MORPHOLOGY

In general, the leukocyte morphology is a reliable indication of disease. In mammalian blood films the presence of immature cells, toxic neutrophils or heterophils, and Döhle bodies are more reliable criteria for infectious diseases than are total leukocyte and differential counts. The same holds true for blood films of lower vertebrates. Immature heterophils of lower vertebrates have increased cytoplasmic basophilia, nonseg-mented nuclei (in species that lobe the nucleus), and immature cytoplasmic granules in comparison with normal mature heterophils. Toxic changes are subjectively quantified according to the number of toxic cells and severity of toxicity present, as in mammalian hematology.[5] Toxic change in neutrophils/heterophils is a term referring to morphologic changes associated with inflammatory diseases that alter production of bone marrow in these types of cells. In response to the inflammatory disease, an acceleration of neutrophil/heterophil production occurs, resulting in the production and release of early-stage neutrophils/heterophils with retained organelles such as ribosomes. Retention of these organelles results in cytoplasmic basophilia and the presence of cytoplasmic vacuolation (**Fig. 14**). Döhle bodies may also be present. Döhle bodies are composed of aggregates of endoplasmic reticulum, and appear as gray-blue cytoplasmic inclusions.

In mammals and, presumably, lower vertebrates, eosinophils are particularly numerous in the peripheral blood when antigens are continually being released, as occurs in parasitic disease (especially those involving larvae of helminths) and allergic reactions (especially those associated with mast cell and basophil degranulation). In general, the presence of an eosinophilia is suggestive of one of these processes.

THROMBOCYTES AND PLATELETS

Mammalian platelets are cytoplasmic fragments (megakaryocytes) within the bone marrow, and participate in hemostasis. Platelets are flat discs of cytoplasm that contain cytoplasmic organelles; they tend to be round, but can vary slightly in shape and size. The anucleated cytoplasm contains variable amounts of small purple granules on Romanowsky-stained blood films. Because platelets are involved in

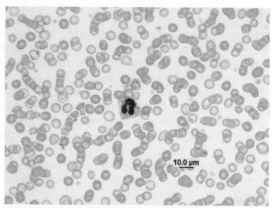

Fig. 14. A toxic heterophil in the blood film of a chinchilla (*Chinchilla lanigera*) (Wright-Giemsa stain).

the clotting process, they are often found in clumps on blood films. Mammalian platelets are much smaller than erythrocytes in the same blood film; therefore, the presence of platelets that are larger in size than erythrocytes (known as Shift platelets) indicate an accelerated thrombocytopoiesis, with early release of immature forms into the circulating blood and an indication of platelet regeneration in some species.

The thrombocyte is a nucleated cell that represents the second most numerous cell type (after erythrocytes) in blood films from lower vertebrates. Thrombocytes are typically small, round to oval cells (smaller than erythrocytes), with a round to oval nucleus that contains densely clumped chromatin. These cells tend to have a high nucleus-to-cytoplasm ratio. The appearance of the cytoplasm is an important feature used to differentiate thrombocytes from small, mature lymphocytes (**Fig. 15**). The cytoplasm of normal mature thrombocytes is colorless to pale gray, and may be reticulated in appearance compared with the homogeneously blue cytoplasm of the lymphocyte in the same Romanowsky-stained blood film. Thrombocytes frequently contain 1 or more distinct eosinophilic (specific) granules located in one area of the cytoplasm. Like mammalian platelets, thrombocytes are frequently found in clumps on the blood film.

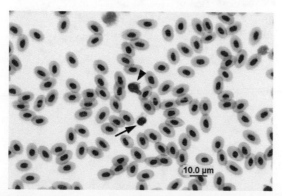

Fig. 15. A small lymphocyte (*arrowhead*) and thrombocyte (*arrow*) in the blood film of a domestic chicken (*Gallus gallus domesticus*) (Wright-Giemsa stain).

BLOOD PARASITES OF BIRDS

Parasites in the genera *Haemoproteus, Plasmodium,* and *Leukocytozoon,* and microfilaria of filarial nematodes are commonly found in avian blood films. Microfilarial nematodes are typically found between the cells. *Haemoproteus, Plasmodium,* and *Leukocytozoon* produce merozoites that invade erythrocytes, and their gametocytes are found within the erythrocyte. Most of the species of *Haemoproteus* and *Leukocytozoon* that infect birds are considered to be host specific. Many species of *Plasmodium* are capable of infecting a wide range of hosts.[26] Parasites of the genus *Plasmodium* can be pathogenic and are responsible for malaria. Certain species of birds, such as canaries, penguins, ducks, pigeons, raptors, and domestic poultry, are highly susceptible to avian malaria, whereas other species of birds seem to be asymptomatic carriers of the parasite and do not develop the clinical disease.[27]

In general, the presence of most blood parasites in wild birds has no effect on the health of the bird, although combined infections with *Haemoproteus* and *Leukocytozoon* can produce a fatal anemia.[28,29] Birds may be infected with a single blood parasite, or may have mixed infections based on examination of stained blood films.

Haemoproteus only appears in the peripheral blood of birds in the gametocyte stage. The appearance of the gametocyte is variable, and may range from small developing ring forms to the elongate crescent-shaped mature gametocytes that partially encircle the erythrocyte nucleus to form the characteristic halter shape (**Fig. 16**).[30] Mature gametocytes typically occupy greater than one-half of the cytoplasmic volume of the host erythrocyte and cause minimal displacement of the host cell nucleus: the nucleus is never pushed to the cell margin. *Haemoproteus* gametocytes contain refractile, yellow to brown to black pigment granules representing iron pigment deposited as a result of hemoglobin utilization. Erythrocytes parasitized by *Haemoproteus* are larger than normal erythrocytes, which likely causes the cells to become fragile.

Key features used to differentiate *Plasmodium* from *Haemoproteus* are the presence of schizogony in the peripheral blood, parasite stages within thrombocytes and leukocytes, and gametocytes (which also contain refractile pigment granules) that cause marked displacement of the erythrocyte nucleus. Identification of the *Plasmodium* species depends on the location and appearance of the schizonts, the number of merozoites present within the schizonts, and gametocytes.[30]

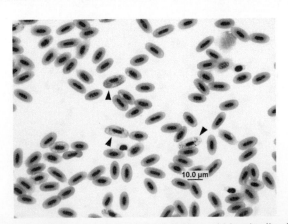

Fig. 16. *Haemoproteus* gametocytes (*arrowheads*) in the red blood cells of a bird (*Colaptes auratus*) (Wright-Giemsa stain).

Leukocytozoon only appears in the peripheral blood of birds in the gametocyte stage that grossly distorts the host cell (presumed to be an immature erythrocyte). The macrogametocyte appears as a parasite inclusion that occupies 77% of the area of the host cell–parasite complex (**Fig. 17**).[31] Microgametocytes are similar in morphology, but are usually 5% to 10% smaller.[31] The remainder of the life cycle occurs in the insect vector following ingestion of blood containing the gametes.[32]

Aegyptianella is a piroplasm that can affect several species of birds, usually those originating in tropical or subtropical climates. *Aegyptianella* appears as a minute parasite lacking pigment granules located within erythrocytes in blood films. Three forms can occur within the erythrocyte[30]: a small (<1 μm), round, basophilic intracytoplasmic, anaplasma-like inclusion; a *Babesia*-like round to piriform-shaped inclusion with pale blue cytoplasm and chromatin body at one pole; and a larger (2–4 μm) round to elliptical inclusion.

Atoxoplasma is a coccidian parasite often found in passerine birds. Atoxoplasmosis is identified by the presence of the characteristic sporozoites within lymphocytes in peripheral blood films. Affected lymphocytes contain small (3–5 μm), pale, round to oval eosinophilic intracytoplasmic inclusions or sporozoites that indent the host cell nucleus, resulting in a characteristic crescent shape in Romanowsky-stained preparations.

BLOOD PARASITES AND RED CELL INCLUSIONS OF HERPTILES (REPTILES AND AMPHIBIANS)

Commonly encountered blood parasites of reptiles include hemoprotozoa, piroplasmids, and microfilaria. Common hemoprotozoa include the hemogregarines, trypanosomes, and *Plasmodium* spp. Less commonly encountered hemoprotozoa include *Leishmania*, *Saurocytozoon*, *Haemoproteus*, and *Schellackia*. In general these parasites are considered to be incidental findings.

Parasites reported in amphibians include *Haemogregarina*, *Plasmodium*, *Aegyptianella*, *Haemoproteus*, and *Lankesterella*.[13] The common amphibian intraerythrocytic blood parasites include the hemogregarines and *Aegyptianella* spp.[33] These organisms are considered to be an incidental finding. Extracellular amphibian hemoparasites include trypanosomes and microfilaria, and are also considered nonpathogenic.

The hemogregarine parasites are the most common group of sporozoan hemoparasites affecting reptiles and amphibians. The 3 genera of hemogregarines commonly

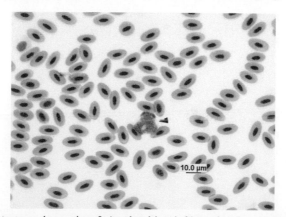

Fig. 17. *Leukocytozoon* (*arrowhead*) in the blood film of a hawk (*Buteo jamaicensis*) (Wright-Giemsa stain).

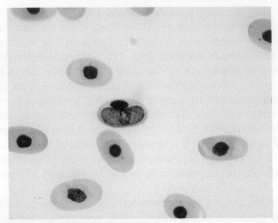

Fig. 18. Hemogregarine in the blood film of a reptile (Wright-Giemsa stain, original magnification of 1000x).

found in reptiles are *Haemogregarina*, *Hepatozoon*, and *Karyolysus*.[34,35] Hemogregarines are identified as sausage-shaped intracytoplasmic gametocytes in erythrocytes (**Fig. 18**). These gametocytes distort the host cell by creating a bulge in the cytoplasm, and are comparatively lacking in the refractile pigment granules found in the gametocytes of *Plasmodium* and *Haemoproteus*. Only one gametocyte is typically found per erythrocyte; however, when heavy infection occurs, 2 gametocytes may be found in 1 cell.

Round to irregular basophilic inclusions are frequently seen in the cytoplasm of erythrocytes in peripheral blood films from many species of reptiles and some amphibians (**Fig. 19**). These inclusions most likely represent an artifact of slide preparation or are considered to be normal findings.

Blood films from boid snakes affected with inclusion body disease (IBD) may reveal inclusions within the cytoplasm of erythrocytes, lymphocytes, or heterophils.[36,37] IBD inclusions stained with Wright-Giemsa appear as lightly basophilic homogeneous intracytoplasmic inclusions of varying size and shape (**Fig. 20**).

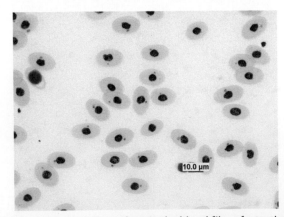

Fig. 19. Round to irregular basophilic artifacts in the blood film of a turtle (*Graptemys versa*) (Wright-Giemsa stain).

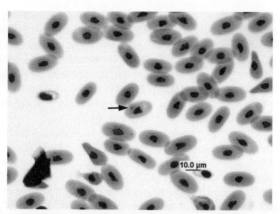

Fig. 20. Inclusion body (*arrow*) in an erythrocyte in the blood film of a snake (*Boa constrictor*) positive for inclusion body disease (Wright-Giemsa stain).

BLOOD PARASITES OF FISH

Little is known about the life cycle of fish hemogregarines. These hemoparasites are found most frequently in wild-caught fish, and probably require a blood-feeding intermediate host, such as leeches, copepods, and isopods.

Trypanosomes are found in all groups of animals worldwide, are usually considered to be an incidental finding, and are not typically pathogenic. Trypanosomes are large, extracellular, blade-shaped flagellate protozoa with an undulating membrane, a slender tapering posterior end, and a single short anteriorly directed flagellum.

REFERENCES

1. Moore DM. Hematology of the rat (*Rattus norvegicus*). In: Feldman BF, Zinkl JG, Jain NC, editors. Schalm's veterinary hematology. 5th edition. Philadelphia: Lippincott Williams & Wilkins; 2000. p. 1210–8.
2. Moore DM. Hematology of the mouse (*Mus musculus*). In: Feldman BF, Zinkl JG, Jain NC, editors. Schalm's veterinary hematology. 5th edition. Philadelphia: Lippincott Williams & Wilkins; 2000. p. 1219–24.
3. Everds NE. Hematology of the laboratory mouse. In: Foster HL, Small JD, Fox JC, editors. The mouse in biomedical research, vol. 3, 2nd edition. Amsterdam: Elsevier; 2006. p. 133–70.
4. Hibiya T. An atlas of fish histology, normal and pathological features. Tokyo: Kodansha Ltd; 1985.
5. Weiss DJ. Uniform evaluation and semiquantitative reporting of hematologic data in veterinary laboratories. Vet Clin Pathol 1984;13(2):27–31.
6. Herbert R, Nanney J, Spano JS, et al. Erythrocyte distribution in ducks. Am J Vet Res 1989;50:958–60.
7. Tell LA, Ferrell ST, Gibbons PM. Avian mycobacteriosis in free-living raptors in California: 6 cases (1997-2001). J Avian Med Surg 2004;18(1):30–40.
8. Wolf T, Niehaus-Rolf C, Luepke NP. Some new methodological aspects of the hen's egg test for micronucleus induction (HET-MN). Mutat Res 2002;514:59–76.
9. Gómez-Meda BC, Zamora-Perez AL, Luna-Aguirre J, et al. Nuclear abnormalities in erythrocytes of parrots (*Aratinga canicularis*) related to genotoxic damage. Avian Pathol 2006;35(3):206–10.

10. Lucas AJ, Jamroz C. Atlas of avian hematology, United States Department of Agriculture Monograph #25. Washington, DC: U.S. Government Printing Office; 1961.
11. Romagnano A. Binucleate erythrocytes and erythrocytic dysplasia in a cockatiel. In: Proceedings of the Association of Avian Veterinarians. Reno, September 28–30, 1994.
12. Hawkey CM, Dennett TB. A colour atlas of comparative veterinary haematology. London: Wolfe Medical Publications, Ltd; 1989.
13. Campbell TW, Ellis CK. Avian and exotic animal hematology and cytology. 3rd edition. Ames (IA): Blackwell Publishing Ltd; 2007.
14. Turner RJ. Amphibians. In: Rowley A, Ratcliffe N, editors. Vertebrate blood cells. Cambridge: Cambridge University Press; 1988. p. 129–209.
15. Pfeiffer CJ, Pyle H, Asashima M. Blood cell morphology and counts in the Japanese newt (Cynops pyrrhogaster). J Zoo Wildl Med 1990;21(1):56–64.
16. Zinkl JG, Cox WT, Kono CS. Morphology and cytochemistry in leucocytes and thrombocytes of six species of fish. Comp Haemat Inter 1991;1:187–95.
17. Saunders DC. Differential blood cell counts of 121 species of marine fishes of Puerto Rico. Trans Am Microsc Soc 1966;85:427–99.
18. Ellis AE. The leukocytes of fish: a review. J Fish Biol 1977;11:453–91.
19. Mainwaring G, Rowley AF. Studies on granulocyte heterogenicity in elasmobranchs. In: Mainwaring G, Rowley A, editors. Fish immunology. New York: Academic Press; 1985. p. 57–69.
20. Filho SW, Eble GJ, Kassner G, et al. Comparative hematology in marine fish. Comp Biochem Physiol 1992;102(2):311–21.
21. Hine PM. The granulocytes of fish. Fish Shellfish Immunol 1992;2:79–98.
22. Arnold J. Hematology of the sandbar shark, Carcharhinus plumbeus: standardization of complete blood count techniques for elasmobranchs. Vet Clin Pathol 2005;34(2):115–23.
23. Walsh CJ, Luer CA. Elasmobranch hematology: identification of cell types and practical applications. In: Smith M, Warmolts D, Thoney D, et al, editors. The elasmobranch husbandry manual: captive care of sharks, rays, and their relatives. Columbus (OH): Biological Survey, Inc; 2004. p. 301–23.
24. Weiser G. Introduction to leukocytes and the leukogram. In: Thrall MA, Weiser G, Allison RW, et al, editors. Veterinary hematology and clinical chemistry. 2nd edition. Ames (IA): Wiley-Blackwell; 2012. p. 118–22.
25. Weiser G, Thrall MA. Introduction to leukocytes and the leukogram. In: Thrall MA, Baker DC, Campbell TW, et al, editors. Veterinary hematology and clinical chemistry. Philadelphia: Lippincott Williams & Wilkins; 2004. p. 125–30.
26. Peirce MA, Lederer R, Adlard RD, et al. Pathology associated with endogenous development of haemoatozoa in birds from southeast Queensland. Avian Pathol 2004;33:445–50.
27. Castro I, Howe L, Tompkins DM, et al. Presence and seasonal prevalence of Plasmodium spp in a rare endemic New Zealand passerine (Tieke or Saddleback, Philesturnus carunculatus). J Wildl Dis 2011;47(4):860–7.
28. Evans M, Otter A. Fatal combined infection with Haemoproteus noctuae and Leucocytozoon ziemanni in juvenile snowy owls (Nyctea scandiaca). Vet Rec 1998;143(3):72–6.
29. Michot TC, Garvin MC, Weidner EH. Survey for blood parasites in redheads (Aythya americana) wintering at the Chandeleur Islands, Louisiana. J Wildl Dis 1995;31(1):90–2.
30. Soulsby EJ. Helminths, arthropods, and protozoa of domesticated animals. In: Soulsby EJ, editor. Helminths, arthropods, and protozoa of domesticated animals. 7th edition. Philadelphia: Lea and Febiger; 1982. p. 689–728.

31. Bennet GF, Pierce MA. Leucocytozoids of seven Old World passeriform families. J Nat Hist 1992;26:693–707.
32. Gardiner CH, Fayer R, Dubey JP. An atlas of protozoan parasites in animal tissues. U.S. Department of Agriculture, Agriculture Handbook. Washington, DC: U.S. Government Printing Office; 1988.
33. Desser SS, Barta JR. The morphological features of *Aegyptianella bacterifera*: an intraerythrocytic rickettsia of frogs from Corsica. J Wildl Dis 1989;25:313–8.
34. Telford SR. Haemoparasites of reptiles. In: Hoff G, Frye G, Jacobson E, editors. Diseases of amphibians and reptiles. New York: Plenum Book Co; 1984. p. 385–517.
35. Telford SR. The hemogregarines. In: Telford SR, editor. Hemoparasites of the Reptilia, Color Atlas and Text. Boca Raton (FL): CRC Press; 2009. p. 199–260.
36. Chang L, Jacobson ER. Inclusion body disease, a worldwide infectious disease of boid snakes: a review. J Exotic Pet Med 2010;19:216–25.
37. Banajee KH, Chang LW, Jacobson ER, et al. What is your diagnosis? Blood film from a boa constrictor. Vet Clin Pathol 2012;41(1):158–9.

Clinical Technique: Techniques in the Practice Diagnostic Laboratory: A Review

Bob Doneley, BVSc, FACVSc (Avian Health), CMAVA

KEYWORDS

- Biochemistry • Culture • Cytology • Hematology • Fecal • Laboratory

Companion avian and exotic animal medicine often stands apart from conventional small animal medicine (eg, dogs, cats) because of the critical condition in which many of these patients present. The "masking phenomenon" that is seen with exotic animals (ie, the natural instinct of prey species to mask signs of illness to avoid predation), along with an owner's lack of knowledge regarding signs of illness in these species, often results in the animal being presented in poor physical condition and requiring rapid medical assessment and treatment.

It is often stated that "necessity is the mother of invention." Consequently, the need to obtain a rapid clinical assessment of these patients has led to the increased use of on-site diagnostic testing by veterinarians treating companion birds and exotic animals. Although this new technology is a significant advancement to the medical services these practices provide, it is not without pitfalls. This article explores the use of on-site veterinary diagnostic testing: advantages and disadvantages of such testing; tests that are performed; type of equipment available; and the need for quality control. Armed with this knowledge, veterinarians treating companion birds and exotic animals can make informed decisions about the level and depth of diagnostic tests they wish to offer, whether to invest in relatively expensive equipment, and how to determine the validity of the test results obtained.

WHY DO ON-SITE CLINICAL PATHOLOGY DIAGNOSTIC TESTING?

Before a decision is made regarding the investment of a machine that performs on-site diagnostic testing, it is advisable for the practitioner to contemplate the advantages and disadvantages of offering this service (**Table 1**). Many of the hematological and biochemical parameters that are assessed in exotic pet medicine can be affected

This article originally appeared in the *Journal of Exotic Pet Medicine*, Volume 20, Number 2, 2011; p. 117–23.
Veterinary Medical Centre, School of Veterinary Science, University of Queensland, Building 8156, Gatton, Queensland 4343, Australia
E-mail address: r.doneley@uq.edu.au

Table 1
Advantages and disadvantages of on-site diagnostic laboratory testing

Advantages	Disadvantages
Sample quality is not affected by transport	Costs of equipment and reagents
STAT testing for critical cases	The range of parameters tested may be
Sample volume required is often small	limited
The tests selected are often more relevant to birds and exotics	Interpretation of the results must be made by the practitioner, rather than by a trained
There is a perception of increased "customer service"	pathologist
On-site laboratories can be a profit center for the practice	Quality control is important—and often neglected

by collection, handling, and transport of blood samples. In particular, hemolysis and prolonged contact time with erythrocytes (**Figs. 1** and **2**) can affect the serum levels of bile acids, bilirubin, lactate dehydrogenase, creatinine kinase, alkaline phosphatase, potassium, calcium, phosphorous, albumin, fibrin, and glucose. Prolonged exposure to anticoagulants (eg, sodium ethylenediaminetetraacetic acid) can cause morphologic changes to both leukocytes and erythrocytes. Any or all of these artifactual changes can affect the clinical interpretation of the diagnostic test results, with the possible result being a misdiagnosis.

Many artifactual changes associated with blood testing can be avoided by careful collection, followed by rapid processing of the sample through a machine in an on-site laboratory. Alternatively, these artifacts can be avoided (or minimized) by the preparation of fresh blood smears at the time of collection. Also, the blood sample contained in the collection tube should be centrifuged immediately after collection, followed by the removal and submission of the plasma without the erythrocytes. However, a larger volume of blood must be collected to obtain the minimum-sized sample of plasma required for wet chemistry analysis: an obvious disadvantage for avian/exotic pet medicine. Some commercial laboratories will dilute a sample that is too small to process in a wet chemistry analyzer, and then adjust the results mathematically to take the dilution into account. Unfortunately, the accuracy of these adjusted results has not been extensively validated in companion avian and exotic animal medicine.

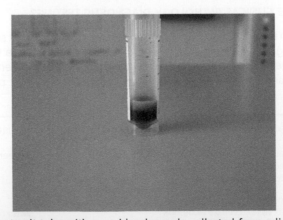

Fig. 1. Microhematocrit tube with spun blood sample collected from a lipemic bird.

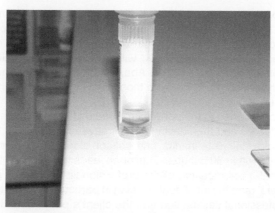

Fig. 2. Microhematocrit tube with spun blood sample collected from an anemic bird.

There is often little time for patient assessment when an avian/exotic animal is presented in critical condition. Many of the patients are severely dehydrated, in a catabolic state, and may have organ (or multiorgan) dysfunction. Although supportive care is essential, specific treatment of a definitively diagnosed condition is even more critical. The actual time it takes to run a specific diagnostic test at many commercial diagnostic laboratories is often measured in hours or less, but transport of samples from a clinic to regional centers and onward to the actual diagnostic laboratory may be measured in days.

The expression STAT is an abbreviation for the Latin word *statim*, meaning "immediately." Used in conjunction with clinical pathology diagnostic laboratory testing, it refers to the almost immediate availability of test results (eg, the Abaxis Vetscan [Abaxis North America, Union City, CA, USA] biochemistry analyzer can give a biochemistry profile in just 13 minutes; and the ESA Leadcare II [ESA, Chelmsford, MA USA] unit can give a blood lead result in just 3 minutes).

Most of the in-house biochemistry analyzers use dry chemistry analysis technology. The major advantage of dry chemistry analysis over wet chemistry analyzers used in commercial laboratories is the small sample size required to run a biochemical profile.[1] Dry chemistry analysis, although more expensive per test than wet chemistry analysis, has been shown to perform equally as well as wet chemistry analyzers, if not better in some cases.[2,3]

The ability to use a small sample size is an important advantage when medically assessing patients that weigh less than 100 g, especially when ill. The knowledge that test result quality will not be affected through the use of a small sample size gives clinicians additional confidence in their assessment of the patient's condition.

Many large commercial laboratories offer a service to exotic animal practitioners as an adjunct to the largest percentage of their business, namely small animal (eg, cat, dog), equine, and food animal diagnostic testing. As such, the experience of these commercial diagnostic laboratories regarding avian/exotic animal clinical pathology may be limited, as evidenced by the biochemical profiles offered. In many cases, analytes are reported that have little or no relevance to the patient from which the sample was collected. Examples of irrelevant analytes reported from commercial diagnostic laboratories include bilirubin or alkaline phosphatase for birds and reptiles. A lack of reference intervals for exotic species is another deficiency of many commercial laboratories. Conversely, on-site machines that run serum/plasma chemistry profiles frequently can be programmed for the species the clinician is treating. Again, as an example, the Abaxis Vetscan machine uses different rotors for different chemistry profiles; one of these rotors is specifically for birds and reptiles. The Abaxis Vetscan software can be programmed as well, so that reference intervals for a wide range of species can be entered and then printed with the results. It should be noted that the reference intervals provided with the Abaxis Vetscan analyzer have been developed for that analyzer and may vary from those provided by other analyzers or commercial laboratories.

Many clients, accustomed to their physician sending them to a pathology laboratory to have blood collected and then having to wait several days to get their results, are surprised when told their veterinarian can collect blood from their pet, analyze it, and have the results within 30 minutes. This often leads to increased "customer satisfaction" and a greater appreciation of the professionalism and skill of the veterinary profession in general (and the individual clinician in particular). In addition to increasing the clinician's professional satisfaction and the client's personal satisfaction, on-site diagnostic testing can become an important "profit center" for the veterinary practice. This profit, however, requires both an appropriate fee to be placed on individual tests and a sufficient caseload to "keep the machines busy." Failure to have either will lead to the on-site diagnostic testing becoming a monetary drain on the practice, rather than an asset. It is the author's opinion that it is appropriate to have a higher on-site diagnostic testing fee when compared with external diagnostic laboratory charges; after all, on-site testing is done for the patient's and client's benefit, and the client should pay more for its convenience and speed.

The preceding discussion is an optimistic view of on-site veterinary diagnostic testing. As with many discussions, there is another side to contemplate, and veterinary clinicians considering the addition or expansion of on-site diagnostic testing are well advised to think about the disadvantages before a substantial investment is made in this technology.

The initial start-up and maintenance costs for on-site diagnostic laboratory machines and associated products (eg, dry chemistry rotors) can be significant. The cost of equipment, reagents, and rotors must be considered, as well as the shelf life and expiration dates of these products. If the clinical pathology caseload in a practice is too low to ensure that all consumables are used before they expire, or the income received will not exceed the loan or lease payments on the equipment, it may be wiser to continue using an external diagnostic laboratory. The decision to invest in on-site diagnostic laboratory equipment should only be determined after careful evaluation of current and future caseload and income derived from both.

Many on-site blood chemistry analyzers have preset test profiles that cannot be adjusted or altered according to the clinician's preferences. The clinician therefore has to accept these limitations, use additional equipment, or send samples to an external diagnostic laboratory. Therefore, before purchasing equipment the clinician must be knowledgable of the limitations of the machine in regard to the diagnostic test(s) and/or analytes required by that clinician.

A major advantage of external veterinary diagnostic laboratory testing is that the test results frequently come with a board-certified pathologist's interpretation. For those clinicians who are not comfortable with the interpretation of clinical pathology test results, this is a major benefit. As the clinician's experience regarding interpretation of clinical pathology diagnostic test results increases, the reliance on a pathologist's interpretation may decrease. However, some commercial veterinary diagnostic laboratories have responded to the "competition" from on-site diagnostic testing by offering, for a fee, interpretation of the on-site diagnostic test results for clinicians who use their own machines.

Another major advantage of using an accredited external veterinary diagnostic laboratory is the assurance that the laboratory has a recognized quality control program in place. This quality control program is designed to detect, reduce, and correct deficiencies in the diagnostic laboratory's testing protocol before the release of patient results, thus having the goal of improving the quality of the results reported by the laboratory. In an accredited laboratory, one aspect of these quality control measures is through the analysis of known samples, which are usually run at the beginning of each shift, after an instrument is serviced, when reagent lots are changed, after calibration, and when patient results appear inappropriate. There would be few, if any, veterinary hospitals that could claim (or afford) the same degree of quality control for their on-site diagnostic laboratory machines. If on-site diagnostic testing equipment is poorly maintained, reagents are stored incorrectly or expired, and some form of quality control is not performed on a periodic basis, the reliability of the test results obtained from this hospital should be called into question. Clinicians contemplating adding on-site machines for clinical pathology diagnostic testing to their veterinary hospital must weigh the advantages and disadvantages discussed herein before committing to a major infrastructure change and investment.

WHAT DIAGNOSTIC TESTS CAN BE PERFORMED ON SITE?

The type of diagnostic testing that can be performed on site is limited by several factors: type of testing that is required; cost and availability of the equipment that is necessary for that particular test; caseload of the practice; space available for the equipment; and the training and experience of personnel who perform the tests.

Fecal analysis, in the form of wet prep examination and concentration (flotation) techniques, is a simple technique requiring minimal equipment and training that is offered in most veterinary practices. The wet prep examination is particularly useful for the detection of motile protozoa (eg, *Trichomonas* spp, *Giardia* spp, *Tritrichomonas* spp, *Cochlosoma* spp) in avian/exotic patients. Many of these protozoa will die in a fecal sample that is more than a few hours old, or has dried out before examination, making the parasites difficult to detect without trichrome or similar stains. In a fresh sample, the enhanced motility of the protozoan organisms increases one's chance of making a positive identification.

Urinalysis—specific gravity, chemical evaluation (dipstick), and sediment examination—is routinely performed in small exotic mammals, but less so in birds and reptiles. The equipment required for performing a urinalysis examination can be found in most, if not all, small animal practices. It must be noted that not all of the analytes on a urine dipstick are relevant in birds (eg, bilirubin, urobilinogen, and nitrites). Urine-specific gravity may not be a valid test in birds because of the potential for fecal contamination of the sample. This test is also not considered useful in reptiles because they do not have a loop of Henle and cannot concentrate their urine.

Hematology analyzers that are available for dogs and cats are also suitable for exotic mammalian blood (eg, rabbits, guinea pigs, ferrets), however, these analyzers are not suitable to test avian and reptile blood. Because birds and reptiles have nucleated erythrocytes, currently available on-site automated hematology analyzers are not effective in assessing blood from these animals.[4] Although the inability of automated hematology analyzers to assess nucleated red blood cells may change in the future, there are no machines at present that will accurately perform this task. Therefore, the manual white cell count is the most reliable hematologic assay for birds and reptiles. The Diff-Quick (Fronine, Lomb's Scientific, Sydney, Australia) and modified Wright-Giemsa stain are the most widely used cytologic stains used in practice when performing a manual white cell count. Total white cell counts can be estimated from a freshly made blood smear, or determined more accurately through the use of a hemocytometer that has been loaded with a blood sample in which the cells are stained (eg, Natt and Herrick). Repetition and a well-illustrated hematology text[5,6] are essential for gaining the required experience and expertise to competently perform on-site hematology (**Fig. 3**). Until the veterinary clinician has gained experience with this technique, it is advisable to submit samples from the same patient to an external laboratory and compare results with the on-site evaluation.[5,6]

The most significant on-site veterinary diagnostic laboratory development in the last 2 decades has been the advent of compact, economical, dry chemistry biochemistry analyzers. This development has led to a marked increase in interest in on-site veterinary diagnostic laboratory testing. There are many different dry chemistry biochemistry analyzers commercially available for veterinary use, and although many use different technologies they all provide comprehensive biochemistry profiles.

As in mammals, electrolyte levels are useful when assessing a patient's fluid and electrolyte status, and can be an invaluable benefit when formulating a parenteral fluid therapy regimen. Electrolyte levels should be evaluated with the understanding of the patient's appetite and hydration status, previous or current therapy, and concurrent disease processes (eg, gastrointestinal, renal), all of which may alter electrolyte concentrations.[7]

On-site serologic testing is a growing field in small animal medicine, but has yet to be fully explored in avian and exotic pet medicine. An avian *Chlamydophila psittaci* serologic test (ImmunoComb; Biogal Galed Labs, Kibbutz Galed, Israel) is widely used in European and Australian veterinary practices; however, as a qualitative serologic test, it must be interpreted with caution (**Fig. 4**). An antigen enzyme-linked immunosorbent assay (ELISA) test for *Chlamydia trachomatis* (Clearview *Chlamydia*; Alere Australia, Queensland, Australia) is occasionally used by veterinarians as a tool for diagnosing chlamydiosis. The high incidence of false positives for avian chlamydiosis when the Clearview *Chlamydia* ELISA test is used on fecal samples again requires caution by the veterinarian when assessing the results. There are very few on-site veterinary serologic diagnostic tests currently available for companion exotic animals.

Similar to complete blood counts, cytology is frequently performed on site in veterinary practices that see companion exotic patients. Again, similar to the preparation of

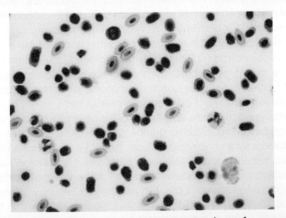

Fig. 3. Experience and expertise are essential to competently perform on-site hematology, as with assessing this blood smear of a sulfur-crested cockatoo diagnosed with psittacine beak and feather disease (circovirus)–induced regenerative anemia.

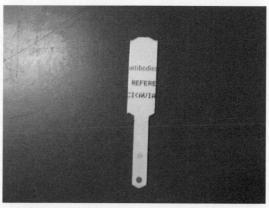

Fig. 4. Immunocomb test used to diagnose avian chlamydiosis. The results from this test should be interpreted with caution.

hematology slides, cytologic sample preparation frequently uses readily available stains (eg, Diff-Quick). Repetition, experience, and a good reference text are needed to become proficient when assessing cytologic samples. When more advanced staining methods are required (eg, Ziehl-Neelsen [acid fast]), a commercial veterinary diagnostic laboratory should be used unless the clinician has a particular interest in cytology.

Bacterial and fungal cultures and sensitivity testing are rarely performed on site because of the multifaceted nature of avian and reptile bacteria and fungi, and the subsequent complexity of the equipment and reagents needed to accurately culture and identify potential pathogens. There are also health and safety concerns regarding hospital personnel associated with culturing potential zoonotic organisms (*Salmonella* spp). Few veterinary practices are equipped, or technical personnel properly trained, to safely handle zoonotic pathogens. If a practice has an existing microbiological laboratory, it is advisable to seek the advice of a clinical microbiologist to develop the appropriate techniques to safely culture and identify potential pathogens (**Fig. 5**).

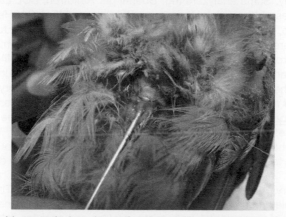

Fig. 5. It is advisable to seek the advice of a clinical microbiologist to develop the appropriate techniques to safely culture and identify pathogens that may be isolated from birds, as with this cloacal swab.

Other diagnostic testing, such as Gram stains and blood lead testing (using the ESA LeadCare II unit), is easily performed on site. However, as mentioned previously, before any diagnostic test is offered by the veterinary hospital, a cost/benefit analysis of that test must be performed, incorporating current and future caseload and equipment investment.

EQUIPMENT REQUIRED FOR AN ON-SITE VETERINARY DIAGNOSTIC LABORATORY

Listed below are some requirements needed to establish an effective and efficient on-site veterinary diagnostic laboratory.

- Adequate space is required for an on-site veterinary diagnostic laboratory. This space should be dedicated to the laboratory; some of the equipment used is delicate and will not withstand frequent moving. The equipment must be easily cleaned and maintained in a controlled environment: conditions that are too hot, too cold, or too dusty will cause equipment failure. A small refrigerator for storing reagents is essential.
- A good microscope is often overlooked, but in most busy veterinary practices is the most frequently used piece of equipment. Wherever possible, clinicians should purchase the best quality microscope they can afford, look after it, and upgrade when possible.
- A staining bench and Coplin jars are useful for cytologic and Gram stains. Staining reagents are often messy, and provision for spills should be made when planning an on-site diagnostic laboratory.
- Gram and Diff-Quick stains are the 2 basic stains most practitioners will use on site. Other stains can be used if the practitioner has a particular interest in cytology; otherwise, most cytology samples should be sent to an external veterinary diagnostic laboratory for evaluation by an experienced board-certified pathologist.
- Hematology analyzers, such as the Vetscan HM5, can be used for small exotic mammals but are of little or no value for birds and reptiles.
- A biochemistry analyzer is one of the biggest on-site diagnostic laboratory investments a veterinary practice will make. Once the financial decision has been made to purchase a biochemistry analyzer, the next decision is which machine to buy. Some analyzers (eg, Boehringer Reflotron; BCL Ltd, Sussex, UK; Idexx VetTest; Idexx Laboratories, Inc, Westbrook, ME, USA; Heska Dri-Chem; Heska Corp, Loveland, CO, USA) use individual strips or slides for single chemistries, whereas others (eg, Vetscan i-STAT; Abbott, Princeton, NJ, USA) use preloaded rotors or slides with multiple tests loaded as a profile. Some of the single-test analyzers (eg, Idexx VetTest, Heska Dri-Chem) can run profiles or single tests. These analyzers confer great flexibility on the veterinary clinician in the selection of test profiles, but require a larger plasma or serum sample size. The biochemistry analytes most useful in avian and reptile medicine include creatinine kinase, aspartate aminotransferase, bile acids, uric acid, glucose, calcium, phosphorus, and total protein. Less important, but occasionally useful analytes include amylase, blood urea nitrogen, glutamate dehydrogenase, cholesterol, and γ-glutamyl transferase. For small exotic mammals, the biochemistry profiles used for dogs and cats are appropriate. The biochemistry analyzer selected by the veterinary clinician treating exotic animal patients must be capable of running the biochemistry profiles and analytes listed here.
- The in-house Immunocomb *Chlamydophila psittaci* ELISA is a relatively inexpensive test for the practice to purchase from the manufacturer, and does not require

additional equipment or extensive training to use. However, this test does require 2 hours to process (if using whole blood), so labor must be considered when determining the price a client is charged.

QUALITY CONTROL

As mentioned previously, veterinary diagnostic laboratory quality control is designed to detect, reduce, and correct deficiencies in a laboratory's internal analytical process before the release of patient results to improve the quality of the results reported by the laboratory. Quality control is a measure of precision or how well the measurement system reproduces the same result over time and under varying operating conditions. Unfortunately, many on-site diagnostic laboratories overlook or neglect quality control measures.

Quality control is more than just keeping equipment clean and well maintained. It is important that comparisons are made between the results obtained from an on-site diagnostic laboratory and a known result obtained elsewhere. These comparisons can be facilitated in one of two ways: either by testing identical samples from a patient in both the on-site diagnostic laboratory and an external veterinary diagnostic laboratory, or by on-site testing of a control sample with known analyte values. Either approach allows a comparison of a test sample with a control sample. Depending on the caseload of the on-site diagnostic laboratory, this quality control practice may need to be performed weekly, every 2 weeks, or monthly. One must remember that many commercial veterinary diagnostic laboratories perform these quality control measures at least once a day. The cost of running quality control samples should be considered part of the operating expenses of an on-site diagnostic laboratory, and should be taken into account when developing a fee schedule for that laboratory.

SUMMARY

Although a strong case can be made against the development of extensive on-site diagnostic testing in a "standard" small animal veterinary practice, this case is based on the expense of running nonurgent samples internally versus sending them to a commercial veterinary diagnostic laboratory. The same is not always true regarding a veterinary practice that treats exotic animals, where many patients are presented critically ill, and time delays in obtaining test results can be a major factor in assessing the patient's condition and determining treatment strategies.

Practitioners considering implementing on-site diagnostic laboratory testing must consider the caseload they are seeing—the number and type of patients—and whether this caseload can financially support the expense of on-site diagnostic equipment. If so, they then need to consider what tests they want to offer their clientele, and what equipment is commercially available to make this happen.

Once the decision has been made to purchase the equipment, consideration then needs to be given to staff training to operate the equipment, staff time when operating the equipment, and quality control measures. Taking all of these costs into consideration, and the client/patient benefits from STAT testing, a realistic fee schedule can be developed to see if on-site diagnostic testing is a profitable operation for that particular avian and exotic veterinary practice.

REFERENCES

1. Hochleithner M. Evaluation of two dry chemistry systems in pet bird medicine. Assoc Avian Vet Today 1988;2:18–23.

2. Bürgi W, Briner M, Aumer B. Dry chemistry in the clinical laboratory: how reliable is it? Schweiz Med Wochenschr 1992;122(51–52):1980–4 [in German].
3. Lopes-Pereira CM, Harun M, Schmidtova D, et al. Use of the dry chemistry "Reflotron" blood analyzer under outdoor-field conditions in veterinary medicine. Eur J Clin Chem Clin Biochem 1996;34:3–35.
4. Lilliehook I, Wall H, Tauson R, et al. Differential leukocyte counts determined in chicken blood using the Cell-Dyn 3500. Vet Clin Pathol 2004;33(3):133–8.
5. Campbell TW, Ellis CK. Avian and exotic animal hematology and cytology. 3rd edition. Ames (IA): Blackwell Publishing; 2007.
6. Clark P, Boardman W, Raidal S. Atlas of clinical avian hematology. Oxford (United Kingdom): Wiley-Blackwell; 2009.
7. Jones MP. Avian clinical pathology I and II. Proc Western Veterinary Conference. Las Vegas (NV): 2004. Available at: http://www.vin.com/Members/Proceedings/Proceedings.plx?CID=wvc2004&PID=pr05757&O=VIN. Accessed September 10, 2010.

Automated In-Clinic Hematology Instruments for Small Animal Practitioners: What is Available, What Can They Really Do, and How Do I Make a Choice?

Elizabeth G. Welles, DVM, PhD

KEYWORDS

* Hematology * CBC * In-clinic hematology analyzers

WHAT IS AVAILABLE?

Instruments with 3 different methods of cell counting, or a combination of methods, are available and reasonably priced for purchase by individual or small groups of practitioners. These methods are quantitative buffy coat analysis, impedance analysis, and flow-cytometric analysis.

Quantitative Buffy Coat Analysis

An instrument based on quantitative buffy coat (QBC) analysis was the first in-clinic instrument available to veterinary practitioners; unfortunately, it is the least automated, provides the least number of analytes, and is the least accurate. The QBC Vet Auto-Read is made by IDEXX Laboratories (Westbrook, ME, USA). This instrument is only semiautomated; it requires several manual steps, which are potential sources for the introduction of human errors. To perform counts and classify cell types, a person must draw blood into a specific tube by use of a dedicated pipetter, cap the tube, place a plastic float into the tube after mixing blood with a dye on the tube's interior, and properly load the tubes in a dedicated centrifuge. The principle of cell counting by the QBC is that after high-speed centrifugation of whole anticoagulated blood in a tube slightly longer and fatter than a typical microhematocrit tube, cells settle out in

This article originally appeared in Veterinary Clinics of North America: Small Animal Practice, Volume 42, Number 1, 2012.
The author has nothing to disclose.
Department of Pathobiology, Auburn University, 171 Greene Hall, Auburn, AL 36849-5519, USA
E-mail address: welleeg@auburn.edu

layers based on their density. This process is called differential centrifugation.[1,2] In order of greatest (bottom of the tube) to lowest (top of the tube) density, the cells layer in this order: erythrocytes, granulocytes, monocytes and lymphocytes, platelets, and then plasma. Leukocytes and platelets together constitute the buffy coat, which should never be used via direct visualization to estimate a total white count or platelet count. With QBC analysis, a small cylindrical plastic float with similar density as the buffy coat is placed in the tube prior to centrifugation. The float migrates to the area of the buffy coat during centrifugation and by displacement of cell-containing fluid around the float the buffy coat is expanded such that the length of each layer can be used to quantify the numbers of cells. A dye, acridine orange, coats the inside of each tube and binds to DNA, RNA, and lipoproteins in cells, which facilitates cell layer measurement via fluorescence with exposure to ultraviolet light. The automated reader of the samples determines changes in cell types by abrupt changes in fluorescence (slope) and produces a printout with analyte information in three different formats: as numbers (such as hematocrit, total white blood cells, WBC/μL, etc), as bars on an "idiot chart" that designate low, normal or high, and as a graph called a buffy coat analysis. The QBC does not provide a complete differential. Rather, the lymphocytes are grouped with monocytes and eosinophils are grouped with neutrophils (as granulocytes). In canine samples, eosinophil counts will be displayed separately from neutrophils if the eosinophils are a significant population within the leukocytes.

The QBC analyzer requires little or no maintenance. There is a calibration rod (painted metal rod) that should be run daily, but there are no real control materials available that can be run to allow the practitioner sufficient confidence that the results provided by the instrument are as accurate as possible. The sample run time is approximately 7 minutes (centrifugation and tube scanning/analysis). Evaluation of peripheral blood smears for cell morphology and verification of generated data should still be part of the routine CBC analysis.

Impedance Technology

Impedance technology–based instruments are the most numerous. These instruments are real workhorses with high reliability and dependability, fast sample cycle time, and high accuracy. They are relatively inexpensive to operate and have moderate in-house repair capabilities if you are willing to learn. Several instruments are available from different manufacturers including, but not limited to, Vet Scan®HM II and HM V (Abaxis North America, Union City, CA, USA), scil Vet abc, scil Vet abc Plus, and scil Vet Focus 5 hematology analyzers (scil Animal Care Company, Gurnee, IL, USA), CBC-Diff and HemaTrue (Heska Corporation, Loveland, CO, USA), and Hemavet 950, Hemavet 950LV, Hemavet 950FS, and Hemavet 1700 (Drew Scientific Inc, Oxford, CT, USA). Each instrument has its own somewhat different bells and whistles, but essentially they are quite similar. These instruments can count and size cells. The principle of cell counting[1] is that cells proceed in single-cell fashion after dilution through a small aperture on either side of which are electrodes and between which a small electrical current flows. The cells moving through the aperture change the electrical impedance between electrodes and produce a voltage pulse that can be measured. Cells are enumerated by the numbers of generated voltage pulses within a designated time frame and cell size is proportional to the degree of voltage change. Leukocytes are enumerated after a solution is added to lyse erythrocytes. Differentiation of leukocyte types and platelets from erythrocytes is based on size as determined by magnitude of the change in voltage. Some manufacturer differences involve use of various lysing agents to which different cells show varying degrees of susceptibility to lyse, which helps distinguish cell types, while others use patented flow technology and software (Drew Scientific Inc has Focused Flow[R] technology)[3] for cell separation and categorization.

Impedance type counters use small volumes of anticoagulated blood (12 to 125 μL) and most have means of analyzing very small (12 to 25 μL) samples (micro-sample system for Heska instruments and predilution setting with Abaxis) when only very small sample volume is available, either because the patient is extremely small (such as mice, kittens, puppies), is very anemic, is dehydrated, or is uncooperative. Any size blood tube or syringe containing anticoagulant can be used.

Impedance type counters typically require minimal maintenance. The instruments automatically self-clean at specified intervals—6, 12, or 24 hours—which varies by instrument. Some require that a blank be used to test the background counts in the fluidics systems (Abaxis). The sample run times are short, typically between 1 and 3 minutes. The instruments have variable capacity for data storage. Liquid external control samples are available from manufacturers and should be used on a regular basis; daily prior to any patient samples are analyzed is best.

Flow Cytometric Analysis

The principle of flow-cytometry[1,2] is that micro-droplets of diluent containing single cells pass into a chamber through which a laser beam of light is shined. The absorption and scatter of the light after striking each cell are measured as forward angle scatter or side angle scatter. The diameter of each cell is determined by how long it takes to traverse the beam of light. Forward angle scatter (low) is used to count and size cells. Forward angle scatter (high) assesses the complexity of each cell and wide angle (right angle) scatter is affected by nuclear and internal cytoplasmic structures (granularity) and is used to differentiate leukocyte types and platelets from erythrocytes.

The LaserCyte made by IDEXX Laboratories is a flow-cytometry–based instrument. It is fully automated, which includes closed tube sampling to avoid sample contamination or spillage and within-instrument sample mixing (all instrument sample handling occurs beneath a cover and is not visualized by the user). For each sample the instrument uses individual tubes of reagent that contain tiny beads (qualiBeads[R]) that serve as internal controls in each sample run and across runs to assess that there has been correct pipetting and laser performance; however, there are no external control materials available for use as quality control samples. The instrument requires no daily maintenance owing to use of the qualiBeads[R], but the beads are not cells and cannot replace the use of external liquid controls. The instrument cycle time is quite long; results are provided in approximately 8 to 10 minutes and then the instrument continues cleaning itself for 5 to 7 additional minutes. And there are very limited to no means of performing any in-house troubleshooting.

The ProCyte Dx by IDEXX Laboratories utilizes a combination of flow-cytometric, optical fluorescence, and impedance analysis to count and differentiate cells.[2] Impedance technology is used to analyze erythrocytes, flow-cytometry and fluorescence are used to count leukocytes and perform leukocyte differential counts, and optical fluorescence is used to perform reticulocyte and platelet counts. The optical fluorescence analysis of cells eliminates interference between large erythrocytes and clumped platelets and provides additional specificity for analysis of leukocytes. External liquid quality controls are available.

As with the LaserCyte, the ProCyte Dx requires no sample preparation after proper collection of blood into specialized EDTA-containing tubes and seven or eight inversions to ensure proper mixing of blood with anticoagulant. There is closed tube sampling and on-board sample mixing. Sample cycle time is 2 minutes for the ProCyte Dx.

The IDEXX LaserCyte and ProCyte Dx use special blood tubes called IDEXX Vet-Collect[R] tubes. These tubes contain EDTA and are the size of a typical 5-mL sample draw tube, but they are intended to hold only 0.5 to 1.5 mL of whole blood. Although each instrument requires a small sample (95 or 30 μL for LaserCyte or ProCyte Dx, respectively), the instrument automated sampling system will not function properly if less than 0.5 mL or more than 1.5 mL of blood is present in the tubes.

WHAT CAN IN-CLINIC HEMATOLOGY INSTRUMENTS REALLY DO?

The IDEXX QBC provides the least CBC analytes (**Table 1**) and has the least accuracy of the various instruments based on results from several studies.[4,5] The instrument is semiautomated with several manual steps, which allow introduction of human error. The hematocrit from the QBC is quite accurate because it is basically a spun hematocrit (or packed cell volume [PCV]). The platelet count is provided as the number of platelets per microliter, but it is really a plateletcrit that has been converted to a platelet count. For dogs with macrothrombocytopenia,[6] this method of platelet enumeration (plateletcrit) appears to be more accurate than counts from instruments with other methodologies. The QBC method of platelet counting theoretically should be more accurate for cats and samples with clumped platelets[7,8]; however, this has not been found.[4] Feline platelets are often large and may have size overlap with their erythrocytes.[8] Impedance and, to a lesser extent, flow-cytometric instruments often count larger platelets and clumps of platelets as erythrocytes.[9] Platelet clumping is another problem often encountered in cats owing to the reactive nature of their platelets and because feline patients are often difficult to collect blood from with first-time, clean venipuncture. The inclusion of some platelets as erythrocytes has an almost imperceptible effect on red blood cells (RBCs) because there are only thousands of platelets and there are millions of erythrocytes. However, the patients are often reported to have thrombocytopenia. One should never believe a cat is thrombocytopenic based on instrument-derived values until a blood smear has been evaluated and platelet numbers have been estimated. With the ×100 (oil) objective, there should be an averaged minimum of 8 to 10 platelets per field; this is approximately 150,000 to 200,000 platelets/μL [formula: estimated platelet count/μL = average platelets per 100 (oil) objective field × 15,000 to 20,000].[10] Dogs with macrothrombocytopenia[11] (nearly all Cavalier King Charles Spaniels and a few individuals in several other breeds) have low numbers of platelets (30,000 to 100,000/μL often) that have large volume (12 to 34 fL or larger) such that the "platelet mass," which is typically normal (no bleeding tendency), is better represented by the plateletcrit.[6] Other measured analytes from the IDEXX QBC are less accurate than their counterparts as measured on impedance of flow-cytometric instruments.[5]

The main differences between the available analytes (see **Table 1**) from impedance-based and flow-cytometric/flow plus impedance–based instruments fall into 3 areas: nucleated RBC (nRBC) inclusion in the WBC, leukocyte differential, and reticulocyte determination results. Impedance-based instruments add lysing agents for erythrocyte removal prior to enumeration of leukocytes; however, the lysing agents actually lyse all cells. The nuclei of cells from which the cytoplasm is stripped are counted and sized; therefore, the nuclei of nRBCs are included as WBCs. This occasionally can lead to erroneous diagnoses when numerous nRBCs are in circulation such as in strongly regenerative anemias, in situations of vascular injury (sepsis or heat stroke), or in neoplastic or dysplastic conditions (erythroleukemia or myelodysplastic syndrome-erythroid dominant). A 5-part leukocyte differential is available on dogs, cats, and horses on the Vet Scan HMV and on dogs, cats,

Table 1
Analytes included in CBC results from various in-clinic hematology instruments

Analyte	IDEXX QBC[2]	Vet Scan HMII[17] Vet Scan HMV	Heska CBC-Diff[18] Heska HemaTrue	Hemavet 950[3,c] Hemavet 1700[c]	scil Vet abc[19] scil Vet abc Plus scil Vet Focus 5[d]	IDEXX LaserCyte[2] IDEXX ProCyte[e]
RBC		X	X	X	X	X
HGB	X	X	X	X	X	X
HCT	X	X	X	X	X	X
MCV		X	X	X	X	X
MCH		X	X	X	X	X
MCHC	X	X	X	X	X	X
RDW		X	X	X		X
Reticulocytes, %	X					X
Absolute reticulocyte count						X
PLT	X	X	X	X	X	X
MPV		X	X	X		X
PDW						X
PCT						X
WBC	X	X	X	X	X	X
Neutros, %	X[a]	X	X	X	X	X
Lymphs, %		X	X	X	X	X
Monos, %		X	X	X	X	X
Lymph + mono, %	X					
Eos, %	X[a]	X[b]		X	Flagged if >5%	X
Baso, %		X[b]		X		X
Neutros, n	X[a]	X	X	X	X	X
Lymphs, n		X	X	X	X	X
Monos, n		X	X	X	X	X
Lymph + mono, n	X					
Eos, n	X[a]	X[b]		X	If >5%	X
Baso, n		X[b]		X		X

Abbreviations: HCT, hematocrit; HGB, hemoglobin; MCH, mean corpuscular hemoglobin; MCHC, mean corpuscular hemoglobin concentration; MCV, mean corpuscular volume; MPV, mean platelet volume; PCT, plateletcrit; PDW, platelet distribution width; PLT, platelets; RDW, red cell distribution width.

[a] Eosinophils cannot be differentiated from neutrophils in cats or horses.[2]

[b] Leukocyte 5-part differential available on HMV[16] for dogs, cats, and horses. Leukocyte 3-part differential available on HMV for mice, rabbits, rats, ferrets, pigs, cattle, and monkeys (research). Vet Scan HMII provides a 3-part leukocyte differential only on all validated species.

[c] Hemavet 950[3] offers CBC analysis on dogs, cats, calves, cattle, ferrets, foals, goats, Guinea pigs, horses, pigs, sheep, and rabbits. Hemavet 1700 has additional species including camel, deer, elephants, llamas, monkeys, mice, rats, and pre-diluted rats and mice.

[d] scil Vet Focus 5[18] appears to be identical to Hemavet 950 from Drew Scientific Inc.[3]

[e] IDEXX LaserCyte and ProCyte Dx[2] provide a 5-part differential on dogs, cats, horses, cattle, and ferrets. The 24 listed analytes are not available depending on species, such as retic percent and nRBC values are not available for horses.

Information obtained from manufacturer websites: IDEXX.com, Abaxis.com, Heska.com, Drewscientific.com, and scil.com.

horses, cattle, and ferrets on the IDEXX LaserCyte and ProCyte Dx.[2] The leukocyte differential is the weakest part of the CBC on all semiautomated and fully automated instruments, regardless of the manufacturers' claims.[5,6,12–16] A 5-part differential (neutrophils, lymphocytes, monocytes, eosinophils, and basophils) should provide the practitioner more information than does a 3-part differential (neutrophils, lymphocytes, and monocytes), but the cell types other than the most numerous type of cells (typically neutrophils) have questionable accuracy[12,15,16] and none of the instruments identify band neutrophils. Thus examination of cell morphology on a blood smear is essential for validation of data from these instruments as well as for identification of nucleated erythrocytes, neutrophilic left shifts (band neutrophils or earlier precursor cells), toxic changes in neutrophils, and lymphocyte and other leukocyte abnormalities and for the detection of low numbers of circulating blast-type cells or mast cells. Additionally, erythrocyte morphologic evaluation from blood smears is extremely beneficial in the pursuit of a cause of anemia. Flow cytometry–based instruments provide reticulocyte enumeration, which is quite helpful in determination of presence of regeneration in anemia, especially in dogs and cats. Results of reticulocyte analysis on a LaserCyte instrument showed only moderate accuracy compared with results from an Advia 120 (Siemens Healthcare Diagnostics, Deerfield, IL, USA; multispecies software), an instrument often considered a "gold standard" in diagnostic hematology. Reticulocytes were underreported in patients shown to have reticulocytes from Advia 120 data, and in those where they were reported, they were enumerated at lower values.[16]

HOW DO I DECIDE WHICH HEMATOLOGY INSTRUMENT IS BEST FOR ME AND MY PRACTICE?

There are numerous considerations that need to be made in the selection of the most suitable in-office hematology instrument for any particular practice (**Table 2**). How much space is available in which the instrument must fit? Does the instrument need to be near a sink for reagent disposal or in a cooler section of the building owing to sensitivity to heat or on a surface with no vibration such as avoidance of placement near a centrifuge? Some obvious considerations involve money issues. How much is the initial financial outlay to purchase the instrument? What are the costs of reagents, controls, and disposables? What is the warranty on the instrument and the cost of a service or repair contract after the warranty period? What is provided in the service or repair contract; for what exactly are you paying? I would suggest that you always have a service or repair contract because once you get accustomed to having an in-office hematology instrument you will not want to be without one. Can the instrument interface with other in-office instruments in your practice, such as a clinical chemistry or blood gas/electrolyte instrument? Is report storage in the instrument important to you? How important is the ability of the instrument to analyze blood from multiple different species? How important is the speed with which results are provided by the instrument? How important is it that the instrument has the capability to function with very small sample volume?

Some less obvious questions also must be considered. How is the in-office hematology instrument going to be used? Who will run the samples and control materials on the instrument? Does the manufacturer provide control reagents and what is their cost? Can data from control samples be stored and tracked for quality control assessment? (In the future in order to pass hospital inspections, clinics that use in-house hematology instruments and other analyzers may be required to show quality control records—that is, not just that appropriate controls are being run, but that if there are

Table 2
Selected characteristics of the various in-office hematology instruments

Parameter	IDEXX QBC	Vet Scan HMII Vet Scan HMV	Heska CBC-Diff Heska HemaTrue	Hemavet 950 Hemavet 1700	scil Vet abc scil Vet abc Plus scil Vet Focus 5	IDEXX LaserCyte IDEXX ProCyte
Sample size	~200 µL	50 µL	125 µL	20 µL	12 µL	95 µL LaserCyte 30 µL ProCyte
Microsample mode and amount	Not available	Automated calculations for 1:5 dilution for high values and small volume samples	20 µL True 20 sampling	Not needed, sample volume required very small	Not needed, sample volume required very small	Not available, sample volume required for ProCyte very small
Minimum blood in tube required	~50C µL	~100 µL ~20 µL for dilution	~200 µL ~20 µL for microsampling	~50 µL	~25 µL	0.5 mL (500 µL)
Sample run time	7 minutes	2–3 minutes	57 sec CBC-Diff 55 sec HemaTrue	2 min	1–1.5 min	Results in ~10 min, total time ~15 min for LaserCyte ~2 min ProCyte
Maintenance	Calibration rod daily	Self-cleaning daily Blank for fluidics every 12 hours	Self-cleaning daily	Self-cleaning daily	Self-cleaning daily	No daily maintenance for LaserCyte Cleaning for ProCyte touch button
Data storage	Not available	1000–2000 reports	Large volume	50 reports	300 reports	Large volume
Interaction with data management systems	IDEXX VetLab data management system	VetScan VS2 Analyzer and data management system	Heska data management system	Yes	Yes	IDEXX VetLab data management system

Information obtained from manufacturer websites: IDEXX.com, Abaxis.com, Heska.com, Drew-scientific.com, and scil.com.

problems, corrective actions are being taken.) And, finally, who will be in charge of the instrument care, maintenance, and record keeping?

My suggestions for how an in-office automated hematology instrument would be used are the following. (1) Use the hematology instrument to do CBCs on well patients prior to elective surgery, for obtainment of baseline data on geriatric well patients, or on minimally ill patients prior to needed surgery (such as cystotomy, subcutaneous mass removal, drain placement in abscesses, clean and repair trauma-induced wounds, etc). If the values from all analytes are within their reference intervals, then a blood smear may not have to be evaluated. You will miss a few inflammatory leukograms where the total leukocyte and neutrophil counts are within reference limits (no band neutrophils or earlier precursor cells are identified by any instrument), a few eosinophilias (if the instrument performs only a 3-part differential or even if a 5-part differential is provided, the differential data are questionable), some lymphoma/leukemia cases where the total numbers of leukocytes and the differentials are within reference limits, and a few other types of hematologic abnormalities. (2) Perform CBCs on ill patients, and if they have ANY values outside the reference intervals, then a blood smear should be evaluated by you, your technician, or sent to a laboratory where blood smears are evaluated on a daily basis. (3) Perform CBCs on patients for evaluation of disease progression or response to treatment. Compare and contrast the findings with previous data. These patients may or may not need to have blood smears evaluated dependant on the disorder being treated. Regardless of the desire of many busy practitioners that the in-office hematology instrument do a truly COMPLETE CBC, all hematology analyzers have limitations—cell morphologic changes cannot be assessed by any instrument. A pair of trained human eyes still must evaluate a well-made blood smear! Your decision to have an in-office hematology analyzer likely includes the desire to have more immediate diagnostic data towards disease identification, determination of health status of a patient, and evaluation of patient disease response to treatment. Additionally, the performance of diagnostic testing can offer a means of revenue generation once the initial investment has been recovered. These instruments, with proper care and maintenance, typically far outlast recovery of investment costs even if the CBC is priced fairly low. Remember to factor-in the cost of control materials into your prices; it is all part of providing accurate and reliable data for your clients.

Who will run the hematology instrument needs to be determined. The instruments last a lot longer if only a limited number of individuals have access to them. These individuals need to be trained, which is often a service provided by the instrument manufacturer, and then these individuals gain considerable insight into the nuances of their instrument based on daily use. The care of the instrument is paramount to its longevity. Most of these in-office hematology instruments are fairly rugged, some are virtual workhorses, but all will have longer life if proper care is provided. Cleanliness is next to godliness is aptly applied to these situations.

SUMMARY

To have an in-clinic hematology instrument in your practice and how it is used are decisions that precede the purchase of an instrument. Advantages and limitations of the various instruments should be considered. Initial purchase cost, reagent/ disposable costs, costs of training personnel in the use and care of the instrument, and service/repair contract costs need to be considered.

Once the decision is made to have an in-office hematology instrument in your practice you should benefit from having nearly immediate CBC data results that enable you to provide better quality medicine, more rapid clinical decisions, more closely monitor patients for complications of disease or response to treatment. It should also generate revenue and allow some of your staff members to expand and develop their technical skills as they learn the nuances of a new diagnostic tool and how to provide you with the most accurate CBC information. In the final assessment, the addition of an in-office hematology instrument should improve the quality and efficiency of the medical care you provide patients and generate additional practice income.

REFERENCES

1. Rebar AH, MacWilliams PS, Feldman BF, et al. In: IDEXX Laboratories Guide to Hematology in dogs and cats. Jackson (WY): Teton NewMedia; 2002. p. 22–8.
2. IDEXX Laboratories. Website. http://www.IDEXX.com.
3. Drew Scientific, Inc.. Website. http://www.Drew-scientific.com.
4. Papasouliotis K, Cue S, Graham M, et al. Analysis of feline, canine and equine hemograms using the QBC VetAutoread. Vet Clin Pathol 1999;28:109–15.
5. Bienzle D, Stanton JB, Embry JM, et al. Evaluation of an in-house centrifugal hematology analyzer for use in veterinary practice. J Am Vet Med Assoc 2000;217: 1195–200.
6. Tvedten H, Lilliehook I, Hillstrom A, et al. Plateletcrit is superior to platelet count for assessing platelet status in Cavalier King Charles Spaniels. Vet Clin Pathol 2008;37:266–71.
7. Koplitz SL, Scott MA, Cohn LA. Effects of platelet clumping on platelet concentrations measured by use of impedance or buffy coat analysis in dogs. J Am Vet Med Assoc 2001;219:1552–6.
8. Norman EJ, Barron RC, Nash AS, et al. Prevalence of low automated platelet counts in cats: Comparison with prevalence of thrombocytopenia based on blood smear estimation. Vet Clin Pathol 2001;30:137–40.
9. Zelmanovic D, Hetherington EJ. Automated analysis of feline platelets in whole blood, including platelet count, mean platelet volume, and activation state. Vet Clin Pathol 1998;27:2–9.
10. Tvedten H, Grabski S, Frame L. Estimating platelets and leukocytes on canine blood smears. Vet Clin Pathol 1988;17:4–6.
11. Davis B, Toivio-Kinnucan M, Schuller S, et al. Mutation in beta-1 *tubulin* correlates with macrothrombocytopenia in Cavalier King Charles Spaniels. J Vet Intern Med 2008;22:540–5.
12. Papasouliotis K, Cue S, Crawford E, et al. Comparison of white blood cell differential percentages determined by the in-house LaserCyte hematology analyzer and a manual method. Vet Clin Pathol 2006;35:295–302.
13. Perkins P, Reagan W, Marweg L, et al. Evaluation of the Vet ABC-Diff hematology analyzer for performing hemograms on dog and cat blood. Vet Clin Pathol 1999; 28:120–1.
14. Schwendenwein I, Jolly M. Automated differentials by an impedance on-site hematology system. Vet Clin Pathol 2000;30:158.
15. Dewhurst EC, Crawford E, Cue S, et al. Analysis of canine and feline haemograms using the VetScan HMT analyzer. J Small An Pract 2003;44:443–8.
16. Welles EG, Hall AS, Carpenter DM. Canine complete blood counts: a comparison of four in-office instruments with the ADVIA 120 and manual differential counts. Vet Clin Pathol 2009;38:20–9.
17. Abaxis website: http://www.Abaxis.com
18. Heska Corporation website: http://www.Heska.com
19. scil website: http://www.scil.com

Index

Note: Page numbers of article titles are in **boldface** type.

A

Abaxis in-clinic instruments. See *Vet Scan entries.*
Abdominal vein
    for blood collection
        in reptiles, 66
Acanthocytes
    blood film of, 120
Aegyptianella spp.
    in avians, 131
Age
    avian
        influence on RI generation, 106
Agranulocytes
    in fish, 90
Alpacas
    hematology of. See *Camelid hematology.*
American Society of Veterinary Clinical Pathology (ASVCP)
    guidelines for RI generation, 105–106, 109–111
Amphibian hematology
    blood film in
        of erythrocytes, 121–122
        of hemoparasites, 131–133
        of leukocytes, 126
Analytical error
    influence on RI generation, 108
Analytical procedures
    influence on RI generation, 108–109
Anemia
    aplastic, 119
    in avians, 53
    in fish, 87–88, 93
    in reptiles, 75–76
Anesthetic baths
    for fish, 84–85
Anisocytosis
    blood film of, 120, 123
    in avians, 52
Anticoagulants
    blood film and, 117–118
Anucleated erythrocyte, 124
Aplastic anemia, 119
Arterial puncture sites

Vet Clin Exot Anim 18 (2015) 157–186
http://dx.doi.org/10.1016/S1094-9194(14)00079-6
1094-9194/15/$ – see front matter © 2015 Elsevier Inc. All rights reserved.

Moving?

Make sure your subscription moves with you!

To notify us of your new address, find your **Clinics Account Number** (located on your mailing label above your name), and contact customer service at:

Email: journalscustomerservice-usa@elsevier.com

800-654-2452 (subscribers in the U.S. & Canada)
314-447-8871 (subscribers outside of the U.S. & Canada)

Fax number: 314-447-8029

Elsevier Health Sciences Division
Subscription Customer Service
3251 Riverport Lane
Maryland Heights, MO 63043

*To ensure uninterrupted delivery of your subscription, please notify us at least 4 weeks in advance of move.

Moving?

Make sure your subscription moves with you!

To notify us of your new address, find your Clinics Account Number (located on your mailing label above your name), and contact customer service at:

Email: journalscustomerservice-usa@elsevier.com

800-654-2452 (subscribers in the U.S. & Canada)
314-447-8871 (subscribers outside of the U.S. & Canada)

Fax number: 314-447-8029

Elsevier Health Sciences Division
Subscription Customer Service
3251 Riverport Lane
Maryland Heights, MO 63043

Printed and bound by CPI Group (UK) Ltd, Croydon, CR0 4YY

03/10/2024

01040494-0018